MENOPAUSE EMPOWERMENT HANDBOOK NAVIGATING CHANGE FROM A TO Z WITH GRACE

EMPOWERING WOMEN TO EMBRACE MENOPAUSE WITH CONFIDENCE AND VITALITY

CLAIRE UNDERWOOD

TABLE OF CONTENTS

INTRODUCTION

In the life of each person, stages are linked to their overall development. In women, menopause is a natural stage of changes that are often not easy to accept, especially if they are accompanied by discomfort and concerns. It coincides with the middle phase of life, and at this time, numerous life events can occur, such as the loss or illness of parents, the independence of children, and the risk of the onset of diseases.

Picture this: A woman, vibrant and in her early forties, full of life and dreams, suddenly finds herself grappling with a tidal wave of emotions. The once-steady ship of her existence is tossed about on the tumultuous sea of hormonal changes. She's experiencing menopause, a chapter in a woman's life that often remains shrouded in mystery until it arrives: uninvited and unannounced.

Menopause doesn't mean that you're struggling with old age or illness. Today's woman is usually informed and therefore capable of choosing and deciding how to face these changes. Also, at this stage, she has developed multiple resources and skills that she can use. On the other hand, it carries some risks that must be known to prevent and be able to enjoy this period with full health and quality of life.

But here's a shocking revelation: While the average age for menopause is commonly believed to be around 52, it can strike much earlier, even before the age of 40! Yes, you read that right. Menopause doesn't always wait for midlife; it can arrive like an unexpected guest at your doorstep, leaving you scrambling for answers and support.

But that's not all. Statistics on menopause reveal a startling reality: Around 20–40% of women experience depression or anxiety during this transformative period (*8 Surprising Facts*, 2023). Imagine navigating the choppy waters of your emotional state while dealing with the unpredictability of hot flashes, night sweats, and other symptoms. It's no wonder that 77% of women find at least 1 physical menopause symptom nearly unbearable, and shockingly, 44% of women contend with 3–4 severe menopause symptoms simultaneously (Menopause Support, n.d.).

Now, let's talk about you—the reader. What made you pick up this book? What ignited the desire to explore the world of menopause empowerment? You see, there's always a catalyst, a trigger that propels us to seek knowledge, understanding, and solutions. It's never just the title of a book; it's the deep-rooted need for change, relief, or transformation.

The statistics we've mentioned earlier demonstrate a glaring gap in information, guidance, and resources available to women going through menopause. Are you willing to continue living with undesirable symptoms that wreak havoc on your relationships, work, and mental health? If not, I invite you to embrace the MENO-WISE tool—a tool that will empower you to take charge of your journey through menopause.

Menopause, often portrayed as a formidable and shadowy phase in a woman's life, is indeed shrouded in a thick fog of misconceptions and myths. From its exaggerated depictions in popular media to the whispered tales exchanged among friends, menopause is frequently depicted as a foreboding and desolate journey.

Yet, right here is where the transformation begins. In the pages of this book, we embark on a journey to peel back the layers of mystique that enshroud menopause, aiming to unveil the profound truths that lie beneath. We will venture deep into the tapestry of physiological changes taking place within your body, gently unwrapping the scientific intricacies behind the array of symptoms that often accompany this transition that serves as the initial catalyst for regaining command over your personal menopausal odyssey.

In a world overflowing with an overwhelming abundance of information, it becomes increasingly vital to sift through the cacophony of voices and concentrate on the essential elements. Armed with this newfound insight, you can make informed decisions about your health and overall well-being, taking the reins of your journey firmly into your own hands. It's a journey of empowerment, a process of dismantling the myths and misconceptions that have held you back for far too long.

On the other hand, hormones can be a tricky business, especially during menopause. The roller-coaster ride of estrogen and progesterone levels can wreak havoc on your emotional and psychological well-being. Anxiety, depression, mood swings They all become unwelcome passengers on this journey.

But there is hope. This book is your guide to understanding and managing hormonal chaos. We'll explore strategies to ease the emotional turbulence, from natural supplements to exercise and nutrition. For example, Gwyneth Paltrow, the renowned actress and lifestyle guru, manages her excessive mood swings with the help of her doctor, natural supplements, exercise, and the right nutrition. That's why you, too, can find your path to balance and emotional stability.

The benefits of reading this book are profound. Imagine feeling calm, balanced, and symptom-free for days. Imagine regaining control of your emotions at work, finding intimacy with your partner, and enjoying peaceful nights of sleep without the interruption of hot flashes and night sweats. This book will provide you with the tools and knowledge to manage your emotions, understand the changes in your body, and take action to embrace the second coming of age gracefully.

Before discovering the MENO-WISE tool, I, like many others, struggled through my initial perimenopause years. I tried every bit of information under the sun, only to find myself overwhelmed and frustrated. It was only through practice, experimentation, and the wisdom of a few good friends that I crafted a set of effective techniques and tools to manage my journey.

Now, as you find yourself on this transformative journey with me, I want you to know this is the right book for you. Are you willing to sift through an endless list of remedies that may drain your finances and leave you feeling defeated? Or are you ready to embrace a well-researched, tried, and tested method that has worked for me and many others who walked this path before you?

If you choose the latter, let's take that first step together: Menopause 101.

1

MENOPAUSE 101—UNDERSTAND THE STAGES, SYMPTOMS, AND MORE

Menopause is a term that often carries a shroud of mystery and uncertainty, even in today's world, where information is readily available at our fingertips. Shockingly, only 54% of women can define menopause properly (*Menopause in 2022*, 2022), highlighting a significant gap in our understanding of this natural phase of life. But fear not, for knowledge is the beacon that can guide us through this transformative journey. In this chapter, we will embark on a vital exploration: A journey through the stages, symptoms, and nuances of menopause, a phase that every woman will encounter in her life.

Menopause education serves as the cornerstone of empowerment, the first step on your journey with the MENO-WISE tool. It's the process of arming yourself with knowledge, understanding what to expect, and perhaps even recognizing how menopause may have already silently influenced your life. As women, we deserve to navigate this inevitable transition with grace and confidence, and that starts with comprehensive knowledge.

This chapter is your Menopause 101: A road map to demystifying menopause, breaking down its various stages and shedding light on the symptoms and intricacies that accompany this natural transformation. We will delve into the physiological changes, emotional shifts, and practical strategies that can empower you to thrive during this unique chapter of life.

Menopause isn't just about hot flashes and mood swings; it's a profound transformation that affects your body, mind, and spirit. As we journey together through the pages of this *Menopause Empowerment Handbook*, you will gain a deeper understanding of menopause's impact on your life and how to embrace it with open arms. So, let's begin this journey of self-discovery and empowerment, for in understanding menopause, you'll find the keys to navigating change with grace.

Menopause marks the second coming of age, a transition where you enter a nonreproductive state where you can enjoy the freedom of life, even if that means embracing the joys of grandchildren if you adore kids. It's a phase that signifies the dawn of a new chapter, a transformation that can be seen as a rite of passage into a world of empowerment. However, this remarkable transition is often shrouded in misunderstanding, fear, and a lack of awareness. As mentioned before, only 54% of women can correctly define menopause (*Menopause in 2022*, 2022), and this is not solely a consequence of individual negligence. It's a reflection of a broader issue: the lack of adequate menopause education and awareness, even among healthcare professionals. This chapter will explore the why, the how, and the empowerment that comes with understanding menopause.

Indeed, menopause is an enigma. A significant portion of women, and even some medical professionals, struggle to define it accurately. Menopause is not just the end of menstruation; it's a profound physiological, psychological, and emotional transformation. The first step toward empowerment in this phase of life is understanding why menopause occurs.

Menopause is a natural, inevitable phase in a woman's life. It marks the point where the ovaries cease to produce eggs, and a woman's reproductive years come to an end. It is a biologically programmed event that usually occurs in the late '40s to early '50s.

This doesn't mean it is the end; it's the second coming of age. As you transition into this nonreproductive phase, you are granted the freedom to savor life without the concerns of pregnancy and childbirth. This newfound freedom can be liberating, allowing you to explore new horizons, discover passions, and even enjoy the company of grandchildren if you have them. It's a time to relish your life journey without the constraints of monthly menstruation.

One essential point to grasp is that every woman's experience of menopause is unique. No two women go through the same thing. Menopause's impact is not solely determined by biology; it's influenced by a complex interplay of biopsychosocial factors. Your cultural background, lifestyle, economic status, marital status, family support, education, employment, past childbirth experiences, or losses can all affect how menopause unfolds for you. Understanding this variability is crucial as it highlights the need for individualized approaches to navigating this life stage.

The way you perceive menopause influences your experience of it greatly. For some, it may be seen as a weakness, a loss of their reproductive years, or a troubling period marked by unpleasant symptoms. However, it's essential to recognize the beauty in this transition. Menopause signifies a profound strength, a metamorphosis, and a new coming of age. It's a chapter that, when managed effectively, can bring a sense of liberation and empowerment. It's about embracing the wisdom and experience gained over the years and channeling that into a newfound sense of self.

THE SHOCKING REALITY OF MENOPAUSE EDUCATION

The shockingly low rate of accurate definitions for menopause is not due to a lack of interest or curiosity but rather a reflection of the inadequacies in our healthcare system and societal understanding. Consider these alarming statistics: Only 20% of obstetricians and gynecologists receive proper training on menopause (*Menopause in 2022*, 2022). This means that even healthcare professionals who should be guiding women through this transition often lack the necessary knowledge to do so effectively.

A significant majority of perimenopausal women, approximately 85%, experience symptoms severe enough to diminish their quality of life and intimacy (*Menopause in 2022*, 2022). However, shockingly, 75% of them go untreated and use no menopause management tools. This is a stark contrast to the potential for empowerment and improvement in the quality of life that comes with informed management.

Menopause is not just a biological event; it's a pivotal phase in a woman's life that can shape her future and well-being. Hence, empowering yourself with knowledge and understanding is not just a luxury; it's a necessity. Menopause is a transition that demands attention, care, and preparation. Empowerment starts with education and awareness.

So, why should you care about understanding menopause, its stages, and symptoms? Why does empowerment matter in this context?

Menopause, with its myriad symptoms and changes, can be a bumpy road if you're unprepared and unaware. However, by educating yourself about the stages, symptoms, and potential challenges, you equip yourself with the tools needed to navigate this journey with grace and resilience.

Menopause doesn't have to be a period of suffering. With the right knowledge and support, you can effectively manage the symptoms that may arise, allowing you to maintain your quality of life, intimacy, and overall well-being.

This step of life signifies strength: the strength to embrace change, the strength to reinvent yourself, and the strength to revel in the wisdom and experience that come with age. When you understand this, you can truly appreciate the beauty of this transition.

As mentioned, every woman's experience of menopause is unique. By understanding the factors that influence your experience, you can tailor your approach to fit your individual needs and aspirations.

On the other hand, menopause is a period of newfound freedom, both physically and emotionally. By understanding it, you can fully embrace this liberating phase and explore the opportunities it offers.

This is just the beginning of your empowering journey through menopause—a journey that starts with knowledge and understanding. Remember, menopause is not the end; it's a new beginning, a chance to flourish, and a phase to recognize. In this transition, you have the power to shape your future with grace and confidence.

DEMYSTIFYING MENOPAUSE STAGES: PERIMENOPAUSE, MENOPAUSE, AND POSTMENOPAUSE

To navigate the journey of menopause with grace and empowerment, it's essential to have a comprehensive understanding of the stages that comprise this transformative phase. Menopause is not just a singular event; it's a multi-faceted journey marked by distinct stages, each with its unique changes, symptoms, and effects.

Perimenopause: The Transition to Menopause

Perimenopause is a transformative phase in a woman's life, signaling the onset of the menopausal journey. Understanding it is pivotal to empower yourself and navigate this transition with grace.

Why Perimenopause Occurs

Perimenopause, "often referred to as the *menopausal transition,* is a natural phase that precedes menopause. It usually starts in your '40s but can begin in your late '30s or earlier, and it may last for several years." Understanding why perimenopause occurs is crucial for managing this transition effectively.

Hormonal Changes

Perimenopause happens due to gradual changes in hormonal balance, particularly a decline in estrogen levels. As you age, your ovaries produce less estrogen, which plays a crucial role in regulating your menstrual cycle and fertility. This hormonal shift is the primary driver of the symptoms and changes you'll experience during perimenopause.

Ovarian Aging

One of the key factors contributing to perimenopause is the aging of your ovaries. As you grow older, your ovaries produce fewer eggs, and those remaining are of lower quality, leading to irregularities in your menstrual cycle.

Lifestyle and Environmental Factors

Certain lifestyle and environmental factors, such as smoking and exposure to toxins, may lead to early perimenopause. Maintaining a healthy lifestyle, including a balanced diet and regular exercise, can help delay its onset.

Premature Perimenopause: Causes and Distinction

Premature perimenopause, "often referred to as early perimenopause, is a distinct condition that occurs when a woman completes the 3 stages of perimenopause before the age of 40." It is essential to differentiate between premature perimenopause and regular perimenopause.

Premature perimenopause requires specific medical attention and often involves more significant concerns, such as fertility preservation and hormone replacement therapy. If you suspect you are experiencing premature perimenopause, it's crucial to consult with a healthcare professional who can provide you with specialized guidance and support.

Recognizing the onset of perimenopause is essential for effectively managing the changes it brings. The first sign of perimenopause is usually a change in your menstrual cycle. You might notice irregularities such as shorter or longer cycles, heavier or lighter flow, or skipped periods. These changes often trigger a sense of uncertainty and may be accompanied by other symptoms that signal the transition.

Symptoms of Perimenopause

Perimenopause is often associated with a wide array of symptoms, and it's important to remember that every woman's experience is unique. Some of the most common symptoms include:

- Hot flashes and night sweats: Hot flashes, characterized by sudden feelings of intense heat and perspiration, are among the most recognized symptoms of perimenopause. They can disrupt your sleep and daily activities.
- Mood swings: Hormonal fluctuations during perimenopause can lead to mood swings, irritability, and emotional ups and downs.
- Fatigue: Many women experience increased fatigue during perimenopause, which can be attributed to changes in hormone levels and disrupted sleep patterns.
- Vaginal dryness: A decrease in estrogen levels can lead to vaginal dryness, which may result in discomfort and pain during intercourse.
- Changes in libido: Perimenopause can influence your sexual desire and satisfaction. It's essential to communicate openly with your partner and

healthcare provider if you're experiencing changes in your sexual health.

- Irregular bleeding: Irregular menstrual cycles may lead to unpredictable bleeding patterns, including heavy or prolonged periods.
- Breast tenderness: Some women experience breast tenderness and soreness during perimenopause.
- Weight gain: Changes in hormone levels can contribute to weight gain, particularly around the abdominal area.
- Hair and skin changes: Perimenopause can affect the texture and appearance of your hair and skin. You may notice hair thinning and skin dryness.
- Cognitive changes: Some women report experiencing memory lapses and difficulty concentrating during perimenopause.
- Sleep disturbances: Hormonal fluctuations and hot flashes can disrupt your sleep patterns, leading to insomnia and night sweats.
- Headaches: Perimenopause may increase the frequency and intensity of headaches, including migraines.

It's important to understand that not all women experience all of these symptoms, and some may experience them to a greater degree than others. The intensity and duration of perimenopausal symptoms vary from person to person.

Hormonal Changes During Perimenopause

Hormones play a central role in perimenopause, and understanding these changes is essential for managing your well-being during this evolution.

Estrogen

The most significant hormonal change during perimenopause is the gradual decline in estrogen production, which is responsible for many of the symptoms and changes you experience.

Follicle-Stimulating Hormone (FSH)

As estrogen levels decrease, your pituitary gland produces more follicle-stimulating hormone (FSH) to stimulate your ovaries to produce eggs. Elevated FSH levels are often a marker for perimenopause.

Progesterone

Progesterone, another hormone involved in your menstrual cycle, also decreases during perimenopause, contributing to changes in your menstrual patterns.

Changes in Your Menstrual Cycle

Perimenopause brings a variety of changes to your menstrual cycle, which can include:

- Irregular periods: Your menstrual cycles may become irregular, with varying cycle lengths and inconsistent bleeding patterns.
- Heavier or lighter flow: You may experience heavier or lighter menstrual flow than you did in your younger years.
- Skipped periods: It's common to skip periods or have months without menstruation altogether.
- Painful periods: Some women report increased menstrual pain during perimenopause.
- Premenstrual syndrome (PMS): PMS symptoms may become more intense and unpredictable during perimenopause.

It's crucial to consult with your healthcare provider if you experience severe or concerning changes in your menstrual cycle to rule out any underlying health issues and discuss management options.

Ovulation During Perimenopause

Ovulation, the release of an egg from the ovaries, becomes irregular and unpredictable during perimenopause. This can make it challenging to determine when you are fertile, leading to an increased risk of unintended pregnancy if you do not wish to conceive. It's essential to continue using contraception until you have gone a full 12 months without menstruating, marking the transition to post-menopause.

Biological Changes and Increased Risks During Perimenopause

Perimenopause is accompanied by certain biological changes and increased health risks that require attention and care.

Bone Health

The decline in estrogen levels during perimenopause increases the risk of osteoporosis, a condition characterized by weakened and fragile bones. It is crucial to focus on maintaining bone density through a diet rich in calcium and vitamin D, weight-bearing exercises, and, if necessary, medications to preserve bone health.

Cardiovascular Health

Perimenopause can influence cardiovascular health. The risk of heart disease may increase due to hormonal changes and aging. Adopting a heart-healthy lifestyle, including regular exercise, a balanced diet, and monitoring blood pressure and cholesterol levels, is essential.

Mental Health Changes During Perimenopause

Perimenopause can bring about mental health changes that can impact your overall well-being. These changes may include:

- Mood swings: Hormonal fluctuations during perimenopause can lead to mood swings and emotional ups and downs. You may find yourself feeling irritable, anxious, or even experiencing symptoms of depression.
- Memory and cognitive changes: Some women report experiencing memory lapses, difficulty concentrating, and cognitive changes during perimenopause, better known as *brain fog*.
- Sleep disturbances: Sleep disruptions due to night sweats and hot flashes may lead to insomnia and increased fatigue.
- Anxiety and depression: Hormonal changes, combined with the challenges of perimenopause, can contribute to symptoms of anxiety and depression in some women.

Understanding the complexity of perimenopause is the first step in navigating this transitional phase with fineness and empowerment. While perimenopause can present numerous challenges, it also offers an opportunity for growth, self-discovery, and renewed vitality. By embracing the changes and seeking support when needed, you can navigate perimenopause with resilience and emerge from this transformative phase with a profound sense of self-awareness and empowerment.

MENOPAUSE

Menopause is a transformative phase in a woman's life, signifying the cessation of menstruation and a new beginning. Understanding the nuances of menopause is essential for preparing the necessary tools to navigate this journey with confidence.

Identifying when you've entered menopause is crucial for effective management and empowerment. Menopause is confirmed when you've gone 12 consecutive months without a menstrual period. This marks the end of your reproductive phase, and it typically occurs in your late '40s to early '50s.

However, the transition to menopause, known as perimenopause, can last for several years and often comes with a multitude of symptoms and physical changes. Therefore, it's not always easy to pinpoint the exact moment you enter menopause. It is essential to be vigilant and keep track of your symptoms and menstrual patterns.

Common symptoms during menopause include:

- Hot flashes: Intense feelings of heat.
- Night sweats: Experiencing hot flashes during the night, leading to disrupted sleep.
- Mood swings: Emotional ups and downs, including irritability and anxiety.

- Vaginal dryness: As already mentioned, a decrease in estrogen levels can cause vaginal dryness, leading to discomfort during intercourse.
- Changes in libido: Fluctuations in sexual desire.
- Irregular bleeding: Irregular menstrual cycles, including heavier or lighter periods and skipped periods.
- Cognitive changes: Some women experience memory lapses and difficulty concentrating.
- Sleep disturbances: Hormonal fluctuations and hot flashes can disrupt sleep patterns.

Identifying menopause is not always straightforward, as symptoms can be subtle or overlap with those experienced during perimenopause. Consulting a healthcare provider and tracking your symptoms and menstrual patterns can help confirm the transition.

But beyond the common symptoms, there are often unspoken symptoms of menopause that many women experience but may not openly discuss. It's essential to shed light on these less-discussed aspects of menopause to prepare for the potential challenges they may bring.

- Joint pain: Many women report experiencing joint pain during menopause. The hormonal changes can affect joint health and lead to discomfort.
- Hair changes: Menopause can influence the texture and thickness of your hair. Some women

may notice hair thinning, while others may experience changes in hair color.

- Skin changes: Menopause can lead to skin dryness, which may result in itchiness and a need for increased skin care.
- Weight gain: As already mentioned, changes in hormone levels can contribute to weight gain, particularly around the abdominal area.
- Breast changes: Breasts may lose some of their firmness and fullness during menopause.
- Changes in body odor: Hormonal changes can affect body odor, leading to differences in scent.
- Dental health: Menopause can influence dental health, increasing the risk of gum disease and tooth decay.

These less-discussed symptoms can be managed through self-care and may require specialized treatments in some cases.

The Biological Changes of Menopause

Menopause signifies a profound biological transformation in your body. It marks the end of your reproductive years and the cessation of menstruation, but the biological changes go beyond these visible signs.

Hormonal Changes

The most significant biological change during menopause is the decline in estrogen production. This hormonal shift is responsible for the majority of the aforementioned menopausal symptoms and changes.

Ovarian Aging

As you enter menopause, your ovaries produce fewer eggs, and the quality of the remaining eggs decreases. This is a critical factor in the hormonal fluctuations and changes in your menstrual cycle.

Uterine Changes

The lining of your uterus may become thinner and less elastic during menopause, resulting in changes in menstrual flow and discomfort during intercourse.

Bone Health

To decrease the risk of osteoporosis, a healthy diet, weight-bearing exercises, and medication are crucial.

Cardiovascular Health

As Menopause can influence cardiovascular health, prioritizing a heart-healthy lifestyle is essential.

Sexual Health

As already mentioned, menopause can affect sexual health, leading to symptoms like vaginal dryness and changes in libido. Thus, open communication with your partner and healthcare provider is essential to address these concerns.

Cognitive Changes

Memory lapses and difficulty concentrating can be part of the aforementioned *brain fog*.

Sleep Disturbances

Understanding the biological changes related to sleep disturbances is key to effectively addressing these challenges and risks that may accompany menopause.

What Happens to Your Hormones?

Hormones play a central role in menopause, and understanding these hormonal changes is crucial for managing the symptoms and challenges that may arise.

Estrogen

The decline in estrogen levels is responsible for many of the symptoms you'll experience, including hot flashes, night sweats, and vaginal dryness.

Progesterone

Its decrease can contribute to changes in menstrual patterns.

Follicle-Stimulating Hormone (FSH)

Elevated FSH levels are often used as a marker for menopause.

Testosterone

Testosterone levels also decrease during menopause, which can impact sexual desire and satisfaction.

Thyroid Hormones

Menopause can influence thyroid function, leading to changes in metabolism and energy levels.

Understanding these hormonal fluctuations is essential for effectively managing menopausal symptoms and maintaining your overall well-being.

Your Sex Life Takes a Dip

Menopause can have a significant impact on your sexual health and intimacy. The hormonal changes, particularly the decline in estrogen and testosterone levels, can lead to various sexual challenges:

Vaginal Dryness

Vaginal dryness causes discomfort during sexual intercourse.

Changes in Libido

Fluctuations in hormone levels can influence sexual desire and satisfaction. Many women report a decrease in libido during menopause.

Painful Intercourse

Vaginal dryness and changes in vaginal tissues can lead to painful intercourse, a condition known as dyspareunia.

Reduced Sensation

Some women may experience reduced sensation and difficulty achieving orgasm.

It's important to address these changes openly with your partner and healthcare provider. Various treatments and therapies are available to manage and alleviate these sexual symptoms, including hormone replacement therapy, lubricants, and moisturizers.

Cognitive Effects of Menopause

Menopause can bring about cognitive changes, although these are often less discussed compared to physical symptoms. It's important to recognize that these cognitive effects can vary from woman to woman and may include:

Processing Speed

In addition to memory lapses and difficulty concentrating, some women may notice a reduction in their processing speed, which can lead to challenges in quickly and efficiently completing cognitive tasks.

These cognitive changes are influenced by hormonal fluctuations and may be temporary. Engaging in mental exercises, maintaining a healthy lifestyle, and seeking support and strategies for cognitive challenges can help mitigate these effects.

Mental Health Impact of Menopause

Menopause is not only a physical transition but also an emotional and psychological one. The hormonal changes, coupled with the life changes and challenges that may accompany this phase can have a profound impact on mental health. Some of the mental health aspects affected by menopause include mood swings, anxiety, and depression.

Self-Esteem and Body Image

Menopause can lead to changes in your body, including weight gain and alterations in skin and hair. These changes may affect your self-esteem and body image, which can have psychological implications.

Coping With Life Changes

Menopause often coincides with significant life changes, such as children leaving home or career transitions. These changes can lead to feelings of uncertainty and identity shifts.

Seeking support from friends, family, or mental health professionals can help you navigate these emotional changes effectively.

So you see, menopause is a multifaceted phase in a woman's life, marked by a combination of physical, emotional, and cognitive changes. By understanding this, you can prepare the necessary empowerment tools to navigate this transformative journey with grace and resilience. Remember that menopause is not the end but a new beginning, offering opportunities for self-discovery, self-care, and personal growth.

EMBRACING POSTMENOPAUSE: A NEW BEGINNING

Postmenopause is "the stage that follows the transition through menopause," marking the beginning of a new chapter in your life. It is a stage that stays with you for the rest of your life, and understanding it better is the key to using the tools and knowledge you've gained to navigate it smoothly.

Postmenopause is a time when you've not had a menstrual period for at least 12 consecutive months, marking the end of your reproductive years. Unlike perimenopause and menopause, which are transitions, postmenopause is a lifelong stage that remains with you. Understanding postmenopause is essential as it sets the stage for how you'll live your life in this new chapter.

A Time of Freedom

Postmenopause brings with it the freedom of no longer having to worry about menstrual cycles, contraception, or the possibility of pregnancy. You've reached a point where you can fully embrace your life without these concerns.

With the challenges of perimenopause and the hormonal fluctuations of menopause behind you, postmenopause offers an opportunity to focus on your overall wellness. You can invest time in self-care, exploring new interests, and taking care of your physical and mental health.

While some women may experience challenges in their sexual health during menopause, postmenopause often brings improved sexual satisfaction. You can communicate openly with your partner to enjoy intimacy to the fullest.

Subsequently, postmenopause is an ideal time to focus on your health and fitness. Regular exercise, a balanced diet, and maintaining a healthy lifestyle become even more critical during this stage to promote overall well-being.

Postmenopause Symptoms

Postmenopause is typically associated with a reduction in menopausal symptoms. However, some women may continue to experience certain symptoms, while others may encounter new ones. It's essential to understand what you might face during this stage:

- Hot flashes: While hot flashes often diminish during postmenopause, some women may still experience occasional episodes.
- Mood swings: Emotional ups and downs can persist, although they are generally less severe and frequent than during perimenopause and early menopause.
- Vaginal dryness: Vaginal dryness may continue, but it can often be managed effectively with lubricants and moisturizers.
- Changes in libido: Some women may continue to experience fluctuations in sexual desire and satisfaction during postmenopause. Open communication with your partner remains important.
- Cognitive changes: Memory lapses and difficulty concentrating may persist, but they are generally less pronounced and frequent.
- Weight management: Maintaining a healthy weight and fitness level is crucial during

postmenopause. Weight management becomes a key focus for overall well-being.

- Bone health: Osteoporosis remains a concern during postmenopause, and it's essential to continue focusing on bone health.
- Cardiovascular health: Monitoring cardiovascular health, including blood pressure and cholesterol levels, is crucial during postmenopause.
- Sexual health: The emphasis on sexual health and intimacy continues during postmenopause.
- Mental health: Postmenopause can still affect mental health, and it's essential to address mood swings, anxiety, and other emotional changes as they arise.

Understanding that postmenopause doesn't necessarily mean the end of symptoms allows you to be prepared and proactive in managing your well-being.

While it's common for your menstrual cycle to cease during menopause, postmenopausal bleeding can occasionally occur. *Postmenopausal bleeding* refers to "any vaginal bleeding that occurs after 12 consecutive months without a period." This step can have various causes, including:

- Hormonal fluctuations: Some women may experience hormonal fluctuations that lead to occasional bleeding.

- Uterine or cervical issues: Conditions such as uterine fibroids, polyps, or changes in the cervix can lead to postmenopausal bleeding.
- Medications: Certain medications, including hormone replacement therapy (HRT) or blood thinners, can increase the risk of bleeding.
- Infections: Infections of the reproductive organs can cause bleeding.
- Cancer: While less common, postmenopausal bleeding can be a sign of uterine or cervical cancer. It's essential to rule out this possibility through medical evaluation.

Hot flashes can also persist during postmenopause, albeit with less frequency and intensity for many women. If hot flashes continue to disrupt your life, you can explore treatment options with your healthcare provider.

Hormone Changes With Postmenopause

Postmenopause is characterized by low and stable hormone levels. Unlike the hormonal fluctuations that occur during perimenopause and early menopause, postmenopause brings relative hormonal stability.

Estrogen

Estrogen levels remain consistently low during postmenopause. This is responsible for the reduction in common menopausal symptoms, such as hot flashes and mood swings.

Progesterone

Progesterone levels also remain low, as they do not fluctuate significantly during postmenopause.

Testosterone

Testosterone levels continue to decline but at a slower rate than during menopause. This gradual decline can affect sexual desire and satisfaction.

Follicle-Stimulating Hormone (FSH)

FSH levels remain elevated, as they did during menopause, to stimulate the ovaries to produce eggs. Elevated FSH levels are a hallmark of postmenopause.

Understanding these hormonal changes helps you grasp the reasons behind the shift in menopausal symptoms and guides you in managing your health during this phase.

Physical Changes and Increased Risks during Postmenopause

Postmenopause is a stage that carries specific physical changes and health risks, even though symptoms are often less pronounced. Understanding these changes is vital for maintaining your overall well-being.

Bone Health

Osteoporosis remains a concern during postmenopause. Maintaining bone density through diet, weight-bearing exercises, and medications—if necessary—is crucial.

Cardiovascular Health

Monitoring cardiovascular health, including blood pressure and cholesterol levels, is vital during postmenopause. The risk of heart disease can increase.

Sexual Health

Sexual health and intimacy continue to be a focus during postmenopause. Managing symptoms like vaginal dryness and changes in libido is essential.

Cognitive Effects of Postmenopause

- Memory lapses: Some women may continue to experience occasional memory lapses.
- Cognitive changes: Cognitive function may remain stable or experience gradual changes, depending on individual factors.

Mental Health Impact of Postmenopause

Postmenopause, like any life stage, can impact your mental health. While the intensity of mood swings and emotional ups and downs may decrease, it's still essential to prioritize your mental well-being.

- Mood swings: Emotional ups and downs can persist but are generally less frequent and severe.
- Anxiety and depression: Symptoms of anxiety and depression may endure, and it's crucial to address them as needed.

Weight Management

Maintaining a healthy weight and fitness level is a key focus during postmenopause. Weight management contributes to overall well-being.

It's important to remember that while some of these changes may persist, they often become milder and more manageable during postmenopause.

Self-Esteem and Body Image

Changes in your body, such as weight gain or alterations in skin and hair, can affect your self-esteem and body image. It's essential to maintain a positive self-image.

Coping With Life Changes

Postmenopause often coincides with significant life changes, such as retirement or the empty nest syndrome.

These changes can lead to feelings of uncertainty and identity shifts.

Support Systems

Maintaining strong support systems and staying connected with friends and family is crucial for your mental health.

Hormone-Related Mood Changes

For some women, the hormonal fluctuations that continue during postmenopause can still affect mood and emotional well-being. Seek support and treatment as needed.

Understanding the potential impact of postmenopause on your mental health allows you to address challenges effectively and embrace this stage with confidence and resilience.

Understanding what postmenopause entails empowers you to navigate this phase with self-assuredness. Embrace postmenopause as a time of freedom, wisdom, and a renewed focus on your overall well-being. Use the tools and knowledge you've gained throughout your menopausal journey to lead a fulfilling and empowered life during postmenopause and beyond.

Understanding the stages of menopause is the first step in navigating this transformative journey. Each stage brings its unique challenges and opportunities, and by comprehending what to expect in each phase, you can prepare yourself for a fulfilling and empowered menopausal experience. Remember, menopause is not a destination; it's a journey, and each phase holds the potential for growth, empowerment, and a renewed sense of self.

George Addair said, "Everything you've ever wanted is sitting on the other side of fear." Menopause education can be a journey filled with uncertainty, questions, and, yes, fear. But as Addair's wise words remind us, the most significant rewards in life often lie on the other side of our apprehensions. Embracing menopause education is the first step on this transformative path, one that leads to aging gracefully, living in freedom, and preparing ourselves for the changes ahead.

You've already taken the crucial first step by delving into the stages, symptoms, and transformations that menopause brings. You've equipped yourself with knowledge and understanding, and now you stand at the threshold of the next stage in your menopause journey.

With education as your foundation, it's time to prepare for the change. Armed with this knowledge, you'll be ready to embark on your transformative adventure with grace, confidence, and the tools needed to navigate the world beyond menopause.

Education is done, and now it's time to embrace the preparation phase. This is where empowerment takes shape, where you apply the wisdom you've gained, and where you build the foundation for a life filled with newfound freedom, self-assuredness, and the unshakable strength to face the future head-on. The MENO-WISE tool is your guide, and together, we'll continue to empower you for the journey that lies ahead.

INTERACTIVE ELEMENT: MENOPAUSE QUESTIONNAIRE FOR YOUR DOCTOR

Preparing for a doctor's visit during perimenopause, menopause, or postmenopause is an essential step in managing your health and well-being. This questionnaire is designed to help you gather relevant information and concerns to discuss with your healthcare provider. Feel free to print or copy this questionnaire to use during your next appointment.

By completing it, you'll be well-prepared to have a productive discussion with your healthcare provider about your perimenopausal, menopausal, or post-menopausal experience. Your doctor can offer guidance, address your concerns, and help you navigate this important phase of life.

Perimenopause

1. How would you describe your menstrual cycle during perimenopause?

A. Irregular periods
B. Heavier or lighter flow
C. Skipped periods
D. Other changes—please specify:

2. Have you experienced any perimenopausal symptoms?

A. Hot flashes
B. Night sweats
C. Mood swings
D. Vaginal dryness
E. Other symptoms—please specify:

3. Do you have a family history of early menopause or specific health conditions that may affect your perimenopausal experience?

4. Are you currently using any form of contraception or birth control during perimenopause?

5. Have you noticed any changes in your weight, energy levels, or physical health during perimenopause?

Menopause

1. Have you reached menopause—12 consecutive months without a period?

A. Yes
B. No

2. What are the most prominent menopausal symptoms you're experiencing?

A. Hot flashes
B. Night sweats
C. Mood swings
D. Vaginal dryness
E. Other symptoms—please specify:

3. Are you considering hormone replacement therapy (HRT) or other treatments for your menopausal symptoms?

4. How is your sexual health affected by menopause?

A. Changes in libido
B. Pain during intercourse
C. Vaginal discomfort
D. Other concerns—please specify:

5. Have you discussed your menopausal experience with your healthcare provider before?

Postmenopause

1. Are you in the postmenopausal stage (no periods for at least 12 consecutive months)?

A. Yes
B. No

2. Are you currently experiencing any postmenopausal symptoms or health concerns?

A. Hot flashes

B. Emotional changes

C. Bone health concerns

D. Cardiovascular health concerns

E. Other symptoms or concerns—please specify:

3. Have you had any instances of postmenopausal bleeding or other irregularities since entering post-menopause?

4. How are you managing your bone health during post-menopause (e.g., diet, exercise, medications)?

5. What steps are you taking to maintain your cardiovascular health during postmenopause (e.g., lifestyle changes, regular check-ups)?

2

PREPARE FOR MENOPAUSE BEFORE THE CHANGES

An online survey conducted in the UAE and the UK revealed a startling statistic: A staggering 67% of women lacked the proper knowledge about menopause (Harper et al., 2022). This knowledge gap is concerning because it often leads to women not recognizing the onset of this natural life transition and consequently failing to adequately prepare for the changes that lie ahead. The consequences of navigating menopause unprepared can be challenging and overwhelming, affecting various aspects of a woman's life, from physical health to emotional well-being.

But here's the thing: This chapter isn't just for those who are on the cusp of menopause. It's not exclusively for women in the throes of hot flashes and sleepless nights. This chapter is for every woman because, believe it or not, the preparations we'll discuss here are beneficial at various stages of life. Whether you're years away from experiencing menopause or have already passed through it, the insights, tips, and practical tools in this chapter will empower you to embrace the changes with fineness and trust.

You see, the journey through menopause isn't just about dealing with its immediate symptoms; it's about embracing a new chapter in life, one that can be rich with opportunities for self-discovery, growth, and vitality. Menopause marks a time when we can rekindle our connection with ourselves and our bodies, redefine our goals and priorities, and tap into a wellspring of resilience that has been cultivated throughout our lives.

In these pages, we'll explore the art of preparation—how to lay the foundation for a smooth transition, regardless of where you are on your menopausal journey. We'll cover everything from understanding the biology of menopause to adopting lifestyle changes that can alleviate symptoms, from nurturing your emotional well-being to strengthening your support network. In addition, we'll delve into the power of education and self-awareness to ensure that you not only recognize the signs of menopause but also navigate them with confidence.

So, whether you're a woman who's just beginning to contemplate the changes that menopause will bring or you're well into this transformative period, this chapter is your compass, guiding you to a place of empowerment and preparedness. Let's embark on this journey together, embracing the transitions with grace, resilience, and the wisdom of women who know that change is not an obstacle but an opportunity.

UNDERSTANDING THE IMPORTANCE OF SELF-CARE BEFORE MENOPAUSE

Practicing self-care is an art, a science, and a lifeline that transcends age. Yet, when it comes to the period leading up to menopause, its significance becomes even more pronounced. In the context of preparing for the changes that lie ahead, self-care becomes a beacon of hope and stability, a way to mitigate complications and embrace menopause.

Before we delve deeper into the specifics of menopause preparation, let's first understand why self-care is important, not just during menopause but throughout a woman's life. Self-care is, quite simply, the cornerstone of healthy aging. It's the nourishment of your mind, body, and spirit, allowing you to thrive through life's various stages.

So, what defines self-care? It's the deliberate and conscious act of tending to your own well-being in a way that sustains, nurtures, and rejuvenates you. It involves making choices that prioritize your health and happiness, not as a luxury but as a fundamental necessity.

Why do women, in particular, need self-care so much, especially in the lead-up to menopause? The answer is twofold. Firstly, the premenopausal stage is when your body is in a state of gradual transformation, both physically and hormonally. It's a phase when your system is navigating through uncharted territory, and this journey can sometimes be fraught with challenges. Self-care provides you with the tools to weather these changes gracefully by fostering resilience and bolstering your overall health.

Secondly, self-care should begin before your body undergoes significant changes to ensure you're in the best possible condition. The goal is to reduce risks and prevent burnout and other potential health issues. By investing in your well-being before menopause, you not only mitigate the impact of hormonal fluctuations and physical shifts but also ensure that you are equipped with the emotional strength and physical vitality to embrace this transition.

It's vital to understand that self-care is not a selfish pursuit. In fact, it's quite the opposite. By tending to your own needs, you become better equipped to care for others and share your vitality with your loved ones and community. It's the age-old principle of *you can only share what you have*. Prioritizing self-care is an act of self-compassion that, paradoxically, ripples outwards, enriching the lives of those around you.

THE THREE CORNERSTONES OF SELF-CARE

Self-care, as a concept, encompasses a wide array of practices, but at its core, there are three cornerstones:

Physical Well-Being

This involves nurturing your body through proper nutrition, regular exercise, and sufficient rest. It's about keeping your body strong and healthy to face the physical changes associated with menopause.

Emotional Resilience

Building emotional resilience is vital, especially as hormones fluctuate. Practices like mindfulness, meditation, and seeking emotional support can help you navigate the emotional aspects of menopause with elegance.

Personal Fulfillment

This cornerstone involves pursuing activities and passions that bring you joy and fulfillment. It's about maintaining your sense of self and purpose as you approach and journey through menopause.

With this, you'll be better equipped to face the changes of menopause with strength and resilience. Remember, you deserve to thrive, not just survive, during this transformative stage in your life.

Menopause, a significant life transition, heralds a series of changes that affect women both physically and emotionally. To navigate this transition with minimal disruptions, it's essential to prepare your body for the impending changes. Self-care emerges as a magical tool that allows you to ensure that your body is in the best possible state before the onset or progression of these changes. This is not a luxury but a necessity, especially as you approach this transformative phase in your life.

Think of self-care as an investment, like a gardener meticulously tending to the soil before planting seeds. It involves nurturing your body, nourishing it, and ensuring it's ready for the journey through menopause. The benefits of such preparation are manifold, from reduced discomfort to enhanced resilience. In this chapter, we will dive into the practical aspects of self-care that you can readily incorporate into your daily life from the comfort of your own home.

One of the foundational steps in self-care is to stay updated with your physician or gynecologist visits. These regular check-ups are like compass points, guiding you through the landscape of your health. As you approach menopause, these visits become even more crucial, allowing for early detection and tailored management of menopausal changes. Your healthcare provider can be your trusted ally on this journey.

Hydration is another cornerstone of physical self-care. Drinking enough water isn't just about quenching your thirst; it's about supporting your body's essential functions. Proper hydration can alleviate common menopausal discomforts like hot flashes and mood swings, making it a simple yet potent self-care practice.

Furthermore, sleep is the body's reset button, and good sleep is nonnegotiable. Ensuring you get enough quality sleep is an act of self-compassion. Quality sleep not only rejuvenates your body but also aids in managing emotional and physical symptoms associated with menopause. By creating a tranquil sleep environment and adopting relaxation techniques, you can wake up feeling energized and refreshed.

On the other hand, menopausal hot flashes and night sweats can be challenging, but you can adopt cooling techniques to manage them. These may include dressing in layers, using fans, or keeping a cool washcloth nearby. Staying cool is more than just a physical comfort; it's an essential aspect of self-care that promotes overall well-being.

Moreover, self-care is about identifying and shedding habits that may worsen menopausal symptoms. This may involve reducing caffeine intake, managing stress, and reframing negative thought patterns. Recognizing and replacing these habits with healthier alternatives is an empowering act of self-care.

Additionally, considering weight management is a wise step, especially if you carry excess weight. Excess weight can exacerbate hormonal imbalances and increase the severity of menopausal symptoms. Addressing this concern before hormonal fluctuations intensify can make the journey through menopause more manageable and comfortable.

These are steps that allow you to prepare your body for the changes that lie ahead. With this, you're not only preparing for the journey but also empowering yourself to navigate it with strength.

The adventure through menopause is not just about enduring the changes but embracing them with a sense of empowerment and vitality. One way to embark on this transformative path is to start preparing your body well in advance. Let's explore a range of practices that will help you lay a robust foundation for the changes that will unfold as you enter this new phase of life. These practices, which include incorporating supplements, maintaining a nutritious diet, and engaging in regular exercise, are designed to ensure that your body is ready for the road ahead.

Starting with supplements, these can be a valuable addition to your menopausal toolkit. As your body transitions through menopause, hormonal fluctuations can lead to various symptoms, from hot flashes to mood swings. Supplements such as calcium, vitamin D, and omega-3 fatty acids can help alleviate some of these symptoms and support overall well-being. However, it's essential to consult with your healthcare provider before introducing any new supplements to your routine to ensure they are safe and appropriate for your specific needs.

You have to be aware that the food you consume is not just fuel for your body; it's also a source of vital nutrients that can help ease the journey through menopause. A diet rich in fruits, vegetables, and whole grains can provide the essential vitamins and minerals your body requires during this phase. Prioritizing these nutrient-dense foods can help you manage weight, maintain energy levels, and alleviate some of the common symptoms associated with menopause.

One of the areas of your health that can be most affected during menopause is your bone health. As estrogen levels decrease, the risk of bone density loss and osteoporosis increases. Eating the right foods and engaging in regular exercise can be your allies in protecting your bones. Weight-bearing exercises such as walking, jogging, and dancing are particularly beneficial as they strengthen both bones and muscles.

But exercise is not only about safeguarding your bones; it's a holistic approach to maintaining overall health. Regular physical activity can help manage weight, boost your mood, and improve your sleep quality—all of which can be particularly valuable as you transition through menopause. Aim to move your body for at least 30 minutes each day. Include a mix of exercises that cover balance, strength, and aerobic fitness. Besides, stretching and deep breathing exercises can promote flexibility and relaxation.

While exercise is recommended during all stages of life, if you are well into menopause or postmenopause, it's wise to opt for low-impact workouts to reduce the risk of injury. Start to incorporate these practices into your life, and take proactive steps to prepare your body for the changes that lie ahead. This is not just a physical transformation but a journey toward embracing menopause with a profound sense of empowerment.

DIETARY ADJUSTMENTS

Before delving into the physical self-care habits that can fortify you for the changes that menopause brings, let's pay close attention to some dietary adjustments. Nourishing your body with the right foods can be an invaluable strategy to transition into this life phase with empowerment. These dietary tips are more than just suggestions; they are the building blocks for a smoother menopausal journey. So, why should you consider making these self-care changes, and what benefits can you expect?

First and foremost, it's crucial to train yourself not to skip meals. Regular eating patterns are like the steady rhythm of a heartbeat in the symphony of your life. Skipping meals can lead to erratic blood sugar levels and intensify mood swings and fatigue, which are often exacerbated during menopause. Eating with consistency supports a stable energy supply and emotional balance, making it a cornerstone of menopause self-care.

Reducing or cutting refined sugar and processed foods from your diet is another crucial step. Refined sugar and processed foods can contribute to weight gain, exacerbate hot flashes, and negatively impact your overall health. By minimizing their consumption, you're making a significant stride toward maintaining a healthy weight, reducing the risk of heart disease, and managing menopausal symptoms more effectively.

Phytoestrogens are a group of natural compounds found in certain foods, and they can help reduce the hormonal effects of menopause. These compounds can mimic estrogen in the body and offer relief from hot flashes, night sweats, and mood swings.

Furthermore, it's important to know that certain foods can act as triggers, intensifying menopausal symptoms. Alcohol, caffeine, and spicy foods are common culprits. While you don't need to eliminate them completely, cutting down on these trigger foods can help reduce the frequency and intensity of symptoms like hot flashes and sleep disturbances.

Focusing on a diet rich in whole foods, grains, fruits, and vegetables is a key self-care practice during menopause. A diet abundant in fruits and vegetables can help prevent weight gain, support cardiovascular health, and ensure you get the nutrients you need as your body undergoes hormonal changes.

Menopause is a time when your bone health can be vulnerable, so it's essential to eat foods high in calcium and vitamin D. As hormonal changes can affect your body's ability to absorb calcium, ensuring you get enough of this mineral can help protect against osteoporosis and fractures.

If you make these dietary changes, you're setting the stage for a more comfortable and empowered journey through menopause. These self-care adjustments are not just about physical health; they are about equipping your body to face the challenges of menopause with resilience and vitality. As you take these steps toward a healthier diet, you're making an investment in your future well-being, ensuring that you not only survive menopause but thrive through it.

Preparing for the mental and emotional aspects of menopause before the transition occurs is a proactive step toward navigating the changes with stability. With the right self-care practices, you can fortify your mental and emotional wellness for the journey ahead.

As mentioned before, exercise and sleep are not just essential for physical health but also play a significant role in preparing you mentally for the challenges that may arise during menopause. Regular physical activity can boost your mood, reduce anxiety, and improve sleep quality. Adequate sleep is a linchpin of emotional well-being, promoting cognitive function and emotional balance. Incorporating exercise and establishing a restful sleep routine are vital steps to ensure you're mentally prepared for the journey through menopause.

On the other hand, spending time in nature is a soul-soothing practice that can help you connect with your inner self and find solace amid the changes. Nature's calming influence can mitigate stress, boost your mood, and enhance your overall well-being. A simple walk in the park or a quiet moment by a lake can be a powerful way to prepare mentally and emotionally for the upcoming transitions.

Acts of self-love are like love notes to your soul. Engaging in self-compassionate practices can strengthen your emotional resilience. Whether it's treating yourself to a spa day, enjoying a favorite hobby, or simply taking time for relaxation, these acts of self-love remind you of your self-worth and capacity for joy.

Additionally, journaling is a therapeutic tool that many women turn to around the time of perimenopause. Recording your symptoms, feelings, and thoughts can be a positive way to acknowledge the changes that are occurring. Journaling allows you to process your emotions, track patterns in your experiences, and gain insight into your mental and emotional state as you navigate this evolution.

Practicing gratitude is a powerful mindset shift that can enhance your emotional well-being. Acknowledging and appreciating your body for everything it has done and continues to do makes you develop a sense of contentment and acceptance. This practice can also help you recognize if you need more support from family or friends, or if you should speak to a counselor or medical professional, should that be necessary.

Meditation is another effective way to process the changes in your life. It provides a space for reflection and an opportunity to prioritize your own needs, making room for self-awareness and emotional self-regulation. Meditation encourages mindfulness, which can be a valuable tool for managing emotional fluctuations during menopause.

Last but not least, considering professional guidance is an act of self-care that should not be overlooked. Menopause can present unique emotional challenges, and consulting with a counselor or therapist can provide the support and coping strategies you need. It's an essential part of your self-care toolkit, as it allows you to share your experiences and seek guidance on managing the emotional aspects of menopause.

Preparing your mental and emotional wellness before the big changes or transitions between stages occur arms you with the tools to face menopause. These self-care practices encompass both your physical and emotional well-being, setting the stage for an empowered journey through this transformative phase in your life.

Building a robust support system and gathering the right menopause-tracking means and resources are essential aspects of preparing yourself properly for the journey through menopause. In summary, having a support network in place can make a world of difference.

Building a support system for menopause begins with staying connected with the people you care about. This can include friends, family, and colleagues who provide emotional and social support. Maintaining connections with your current social circle can offer a sense of comfort and understanding as you navigate this transition. Sharing your experiences and concerns with those you trust can be therapeutic and reassuring.

Additionally, you can explore support groups as a valuable resource. These groups provide a safe space to discuss symptoms, share coping strategies, and offer mutual support. Support groups can be found both in-person and online, making it easier to connect with like-minded individuals.

Finding support for menopause doesn't have to be limited to formal support groups. Sisters, mothers, and even daughters who have experienced menopause can provide invaluable insights and a strong sense of connection (*Menopause—Support Networks*, 2018). Often, talking with family members who have gone through menopause can be especially comforting, as they understand the unique challenges and changes you're going through.

Your friends and colleagues can serve as a valuable source of support. Friends can offer a welcome source of understanding and empathy. Hence, sharing your experiences with trusted friends can be an affirming and comforting experience. One woman noted that being open about her menopausal challenges with friends made it *lovely* to discuss hair, skin, weight issues, mood swings, and hot flashes openly.

Nowadays, online resources can be a treasure trove of support and information. The internet offers a wealth of menopause-related websites, forums, and communities where you can find resources and guidance and connect with women going through similar experiences. These online platforms can be particularly helpful if you're looking for information on managing symptoms, understanding hormone therapy, or simply seeking to connect with others.

For more organized and structured support, you can explore organized support groups. These groups may be specific to certain menopausal issues, such as early—premature—menopause. They provide a platform for more focused discussions and tailored support, allowing you to connect with individuals who share your specific concerns.

As you gather these invaluable menopause-tracking tools and resources and build a support system around you, you empower yourself to face the challenges and changes of menopause. Remember, you don't have to navigate this journey alone, and the support and information you need are readily available to help you thrive during this transformative phase.

Exploring menopause tracking tools and online resources is an important step in empowering yourself with the knowledge and support needed to navigate the impending changes. With the help of these means and platforms, you can gain insights, monitor your progress, and connect with others who are going through similar experiences.

MENOPAUSE TRACKING TOOLS

- My Sister's App: My Sister's App offers a myCalendar symptom tracker designed to help you monitor and manage menopausal symptoms. This app provides a structured way to record your experiences and track changes in your body and emotions. It's a valuable tool for staying informed about the nuances of your menopausal journey.

- Caria: Caria is another highly-rated menopause tracking app that empowers women with information and support. It offers a wide range of features, including symptom tracking, educational resources, and community support. With a 4.6/5-star rating, Caria is a reliable companion on your menopausal journey.
- Perry: Perry is an app specifically designed for those going through menopause. With a remarkable 4.9/5-star rating, it offers comprehensive tracking of symptoms, expert advice, and peer support. Perry is your ally in managing and understanding the changes that accompany menopause.

ONLINE MENOPAUSE RESOURCES

- The Menopause Charity: The Menopause Charity is a valuable online resource offering a wealth of information, support, and educational materials on menopause. Their mission is to empower women with knowledge and provide guidance to help them manage the transition with confidence.
- My Menopause Centre: My Menopause Centre is a hub for information, support, and medical

expertise related to menopause. They offer a wide range of resources, including articles, videos, and community forums. It's a place where you can find answers to your questions and connect with others on a similar journey.

- The Endocrine Society: The Endocrine Society provides a comprehensive menopause resource with a map of support and resources. This platform is a treasure trove of expert-reviewed information, guidelines, and tools to help you navigate the different aspects of menopause.

These menopause-tracking tools and online resources are essential companions as you prepare for the changes that menopause brings. They provide you with the means to stay informed, monitor your progress, and connect with a community of women who understand the journey you're embarking on. Empower yourself with knowledge and support as you navigate the transformative phase of menopause.

Jackson Brown Jr. said, "The best preparation for tomorrow is doing your best today." This quote encapsulates the essence of preparing for menopause before the changes take full hold. It underscores the importance of proactively equipping yourself for the journey ahead, ensuring that you stride into the future with confidence and resilience. However, while reducing the impact of changes before they even happen is paramount, it's equally essential to have methods in place to address the physical symptoms you may already be experiencing. This approach to menopause preparation not only empowers you with the tools to weather the changes with grace but also allows you to embrace the present moment, finding strength and empowerment in the here and now.

INTERACTIVE ELEMENT: MENOPAUSE JOURNAL PROMPTS

Keeping a journal can be a powerful tool for self-reflection, understanding, and navigating the various aspects of menopause. Use these journal prompts as a starting point for self-discovery and personal growth during your menopausal journey. Your journal can be a safe space to explore your thoughts and feelings, track your progress, and find empowerment as you navigate the changes. Here are 10–12 prompts to help you get started on your journey:

- What are your current thoughts and feelings about approaching menopause? Describe your emotions and expectations.
- Reflect on your experiences with aging and body changes. How have they influenced your perception of menopause?
- Consider your support system. Who are the people you can turn to for guidance and emotional support during this transition?

- Explore your self-care routines. What self-care habits do you currently have, and which ones do you want to incorporate for a smoother menopausal journey?
- Are there any specific symptoms or challenges you are concerned about as you approach menopause? Write about them in detail.
- Think about your physical health. What changes do you need to make to ensure your body is in the best possible state before menopause?
- Describe your relationship with food and exercise. How can you adjust your diet and physical activity to support a healthy transition?
- Are there any supplements or alternative therapies you are considering for symptom management or health maintenance? Explain your thoughts.
- Explore your emotional well-being. How can you cultivate emotional resilience and maintain a positive mindset throughout the menopausal transition?
- Think about your sexuality and intimacy. How has it evolved over time, and what are your desires and concerns related to this aspect of your life?
- Reflect on your personal goals and aspirations. How do you envision your life during and after menopause?
- Consider your spiritual or philosophical beliefs. How can these beliefs guide you through the challenges and changes of menopause?

3

MANAGE SYMPTOMS TO NOURISH HAPPINESS AND FREEDOM

As we venture into this chapter, we are addressing a specific audience: the ladies who have been experiencing some of the most common and often quite vexing symptoms associated with menopause. If you've been on this journey, you know that these symptoms can sometimes feel like unwelcome guests in your life. But fret not, for we're here to equip you with practical tools and advice to regain control and rediscover your joy.

Menopause symptoms, whether it's the challenging vasomotor symptoms like hot flashes and night sweats or the toll it can take on your mental health, often persist during postmenopause in a significant percentage of women. This can be frustrating and affect your quality of life. However, the good news is that with a greater understanding of techniques to manage these symptoms, you can infuse more joy and a higher quality of life into your daily existence.

This chapter is dedicated to all stages of menopause because effective symptom management is essential throughout this entire journey. Whether you're in peri-menopause, menopause, or postmenopause, the tools and strategies you'll discover here will help you flourish and embrace this period of your life with newfound happiness and freedom. We are diving deep into specific issues and their solutions, providing you with tailored guidance to address your unique challenges. So, let's embark on this journey together and uncover the secrets to managing menopausal symptoms and nourishing your inner happiness.

COPING WITH HOT FLASHES AND NIGHT SWEATS: A GUIDE TO FINDING RELIEF

Hot flashes and night sweats are two of the most vexing symptoms that women often encounter during menopause. Understanding these symptoms and their causes is the first step toward finding effective ways to cope with them.

Hot Flashes and Night Sweats Explained

Hot flashes, also known as vasomotor symptoms, are characterized by sudden waves of intense warmth that can cause sweating and a rapid heartbeat. Night sweats are essentially hot flashes that occur during sleep and can lead to long-term sleep disruptions, impacting your overall well-being.

These symptoms are predominantly triggered by hormonal fluctuations, specifically a decline in estrogen levels. However, various factors can contribute, including stress, anxiety, caffeine, and others.

Certain risk factors, such as smoking, obesity, and genetics, can exacerbate the frequency and intensity of hot flashes and night sweats. Additionally, some medical conditions or medications may contribute to their severity.

These symptoms can have a significant impact on your daily life, leading to mood disturbances, sleep disturbances, and reduced overall quality of life. They can even affect your personal and professional relationships.

Hormone replacement therapy (HRT) is a medical approach to managing hot flashes and night sweats. While it can be effective, it's essential to understand that it may carry certain risks, such as an increased risk of breast cancer, blood clots, and stroke. If you consider HRT, discussing the potential risks and benefits with your healthcare provider is crucial.

Nonhormonal treatments are available, like certain antidepressant medications that can provide relief from hot flashes and night sweats. However, these, too, may come with potential side effects. That's why it is recommended to visit your doctor.

Making lifestyle changes can significantly impact your experience of these symptoms. Maintaining a healthy weight, reducing stress, managing anxiety, and moderating the consumption of triggers like caffeine and alcohol can help alleviate hot flashes and night sweats. Additionally, alternative therapies like acupuncture, yoga, and cognitive-behavioral therapy have been found to provide relief for some women.

FINDING PEACEFUL SLUMBER: TACKLING SLEEP DISTURBANCES AND FATIGUE

One of the lesser-discussed but profoundly impactful menopausal symptoms is sleep disturbances. Many women going through menopause find themselves tossing and turning at night, struggling to maintain a peaceful slumber. The resulting fatigue can cast a shadow on both mental and physical well-being. In this section, we'll explore practical tools and tips to help you regain control over your sleep patterns and find the restorative rest you deserve.

Before delving into sleep hygiene tips, it's crucial to identify any underlying causes that may be disrupting your sleep. Menopause symptoms such as hot flashes and night sweats can certainly play a role, but other factors may contribute to your sleepless nights.

Poor sleep isn't just a minor inconvenience. It can significantly worsen how you feel mentally and physically. The link between sleep and overall well-being is strong. Sleepless nights can lead to increased irritability, anxiety, and a diminished sense of physical vitality. The result is a compromised quality of life during a time when you should be flourishing.

If sleep disturbances are severely affecting your daily life, it's advisable to discuss short-term medical options with your doctor. They can provide guidance on potential interventions or treatments that can help you regain control over your sleep patterns. Thus, it's essential to seek professional advice when sleep issues become a significant concern.

MAINTAINING YOUR WEIGHT AND METABOLISM HEALTH DURING MENOPAUSE

Menopause often brings changes in body weight and metabolism, which can be a source of concern for many women. Understanding why these changes occur and how to manage them is vital for overall well-being during this transition.

Several factors play a role in menopausal weight gain and the decrease in metabolic speed. Hormonal changes, particularly the decline in estrogen, can lead to a redistribution of body fat, often favoring visceral fat. This can increase the risk of health issues like diabetes and heart disease. The good news is that with the right strategies, you can address these changes and maintain a healthier metabolism.

The dietary adjustments discussed in the previous chapter not only prepare your body for menopause but also assist in managing metabolic changes. However, there are additional ways to address these issues effectively.

Creating a calorie deficit, where you consume fewer calories than you expend, is essential for weight management. This approach can help you shed excess pounds and maintain a healthy weight during menopause.

Low-carb diets have shown promise in helping women manage their weight during menopause. They can be effective in controlling blood sugar levels, reducing cravings, and promoting weight loss.

The Mediterranean diet, rich in fruits, fiber, vegetables, whole grains, and healthy fats, has also proven beneficial in managing weight and metabolism during menopause. Its focus on fresh, nutrient-dense foods provides a balanced approach to nutrition. Increasing your intake of plant-based foods with fiber can help keep your metabolism active. Fiber-rich foods contribute to a feeling of fullness and support digestive health. Hence, these foods can be valuable additions to your diet during menopause. They provide essential nutrients, healthy fats, and protein, which can aid in both weight management and metabolic health.

It's also important to keep an eye on sugary indulgences. Reducing your intake of sweets, ice cream, and candy can contribute to effective weight management.

Furthermore, incorporating ample protein into your meals helps keep you feeling full and supports muscle maintenance. Additionally, mindful eating, soluble fiber, and green tea are all valuable components of your dietary strategy.

Finally, limiting alcohol consumption is a crucial step in managing your weight during menopause. Alcohol can add extra calories and contribute to weight gain.

Implementing these strategies helps you maintain a healthy weight and metabolism during the menopausal transition. While the changes associated with menopause are a natural part of life, your proactive approach to health and nutrition can make a significant difference in how you feel and look during this phase. Remember, you have the power to nurture your happiness and freedom through these changes.

ENERGIZING YOUR BODY: EXERCISE ROUTINES FOR WEIGHT LOSS AND A SPEEDIER METABOLISM

Physical activity is not only essential for your overall health but can be a powerful tool in managing weight and boosting metabolism during menopause. By incorporating exercise routines into your daily life, you can regain control over your body, foster weight loss, and enjoy a faster metabolism.

Aerobic Exercise With Strength Training

The combination of aerobic exercise and strength training is hailed as one of the most effective approaches for weight loss and speeding up your metabolism. As women age, exercise becomes even more crucial, particularly during and after menopause. Aerobic exercise helps burn calories, while strength training promotes muscle growth and fights against osteoporosis, improving bone density and muscle strength.

Body Weight Exercises and Gentle Weight Lifting

These exercises are excellent choices for women navigating menopause. They not only aid in weight management but also offer the added benefit of strengthening bones and muscles, making them resilient against osteoporosis.

Cardio Exercises for Weight Loss

Cardiovascular exercises, such as running, brisk walking, or cycling, are particularly effective for shedding extra pounds. They boost heart health, increase your metabolic rate, and help in managing your weight more effectively.

Yoga, Pilates, and Tai Chi

These mind-body practices provide a unique blend of exercise and relaxation. Engaging in activities like yoga, pilates, and tai chi can not only promote weight management but also reduce the risk of osteoporosis. These exercises enhance flexibility, balance, and overall physical well-being.

As you navigate the complexities of menopause, incorporating exercise routines into your daily life can be a game-changer. They contribute not only to weight management and a speedier metabolism but also to your overall sense of well-being. With a proactive approach to exercise, you can embrace this stage of life with vitality and grace, nurturing your happiness and freedom throughout the journey.

NURTURING YOUR INTIMATE WELLNESS: MANAGING VAGINAL SYMPTOMS

Menopause brings with it a range of physical changes, and for many women, one of the most sensitive and intimate concerns is vaginal symptoms. These symptoms can affect your sex life and lead to discomfort. Let's explore the causes and treatment options for managing these issues.

Vaginal dryness, a common symptom during menopause, occurs due to a decrease in estrogen levels. This hormonal shift leads to changes in the vaginal tissues, resulting in dryness and distress.

There are several options for managing vaginal dryness. Medications that contain estrogen or estrogen-like compounds can be effective. These work by replenishing the hormones your body no longer produces inadequate amounts, helping to restore vaginal moisture and relieve dryness.

Moreover, vaginal moisturizers are designed to provide long-lasting relief from dryness. You can apply them regularly to maintain vaginal moisture and comfort. Additionally, oil-based lubricants can provide short-term relief during sexual activity, reducing discomfort and enhancing intimacy. Some women find relief from natural oils such as coconut oil or vitamin E oil. These alternatives can be used as lubricants to alleviate dryness, but it's essential to be cautious and ensure that the oils are compatible with your body.

Menopause may also bring about vaginal bleeding or spotting, which can be a cause for concern. If you experience vaginal bleeding, especially if it occurs more than a year after your last period, it's crucial to investigate the cause, as it could be related to uterine or endometrial issues. The treatment options for vaginal bleeding or spotting depend on the underlying cause. It's important to consult with your healthcare provider to determine the most appropriate course of action based on your specific situation.

Managing vaginal symptoms during menopause is a crucial aspect of overall well-being and maintaining a satisfying intimate life. By understanding the causes and exploring various treatment options, you can empower yourself to navigate these changes with grace and confidence, ensuring that your happiness and freedom are nurtured throughout this journey.

Hair loss, changes in skin health, and other symptoms can be distressing during menopause. Let's explore some practical strategies to manage these issues effectively:

Hair Loss

Hair loss is a common symptom during menopause. To reduce stress-related hair loss, consider practicing relaxation techniques such as deep breathing exercises and meditation. It's essential to manage stress to maintain the health of your hair. Additionally, keeping your hair care routine natural and well-hydrated can help minimize hair loss.

Skin Issues

Skin problems are another concern for some women during menopause. To care for your skin, use mild cleansers and moisturizers after bathing. This can help maintain skin hydration and health. If you're experiencing acne issues, opt for acne products designed for dry skin and consider washing your face with a salicylic acid-based cleanser. Also, using fragrance-free moisturizers can be beneficial for skin health.

These strategies can contribute to managing various menopausal symptoms and nurturing your happiness and freedom as you navigate through this transformative phase of life.

Roger Crawford said, "Being challenged in life is inevitable; being defeated is optional." Don't allow symptoms to defeat you. Instead, overcome these challenges stopping you from enjoying the second coming of age. In the following sections, we'll explore emotional and psychological methods to manage your menopause like a sage with MENO-WISE. These techniques will empower you to embrace this life transition with grace, happiness, and the freedom you deserve.

INTERACTIVE ELEMENT: CREATE YOUR SYMPTOM-REDUCING CHECKLIST

In this chapter, we've discussed various natural ways to reduce menopausal symptoms and enhance your well-being. To empower you in taking proactive steps, here's a short checklist to get you started. Feel free to use this checklist as a starting point to address your menopausal symptoms naturally. Customize it to match your unique preferences, and discover what works best for you on your journey to menopause empowerment. Use these methods as inspiration and create your customized checklist to suit your unique needs and preferences:

1. [ ] Hot flashes and night sweats: Explore relaxation techniques, such as deep breathing or meditation, to reduce stress, a common trigger for these symptoms.

2. [ ] Sleep disturbances and fatigue: Identify any underlying causes affecting your sleep and implement good sleep hygiene practices, like maintaining a consistent sleep schedule and creating a relaxing bedtime routine.

3. [ ] Weight gain and metabolism: Focus on dietary adjustments by incorporating more plant-based foods, high-fiber options, and lean protein. Consider low-carb or Mediterranean diets.

4. [ ] Exercise for weight loss and metabolism: Incorporate a mix of aerobic exercises with strength training, body weight exercises, and flexibility routines into your fitness regimen.

5. [ ] Vaginal dryness: Consider using natural oils, over-the-counter lubricants, and moisturizers, or discuss prescription medications with your healthcare provider.

6. [ ] Hair loss: Reduce stress through relaxation techniques and maintain your hair's natural health with good hydration and a gentle hair care routine.

7. [ ] Skin health: Use mild cleansers, moisturizers, and acne products suited for your specific skin type. Avoid using harsh chemicals or fragrances.

4

MANAGE EMOTIONAL AND PSYCHOLOGICAL CHANGES TO THRIVE

Just as we did in the previous chapter with physical changes, we'll delve into the emotional and psychological aspects of menopause. Like the chapters before, you'll be provided with insights and practical solutions, but this time, we'll be focusing on nurturing your emotional well-being during this transformative phase of life.

A survey of 2,000 women revealed some startling statistics: 69% of these women reported feeling depressed or anxious during their menopausal journey. These feelings are not uncommon, and you are certainly not alone if you've experienced them. The same survey also shed light on how these emotional struggles spilled over into the workplace, making it difficult for women to concentrate and excel in their careers (Hinsliff, 2023).

It's essential to acknowledge that poor mental and emotional health can cast a shadow over what should be a vibrant and empowering transitional phase of your life. We are here to ensure this doesn't happen to you.

In this chapter, we will explore the diverse emotional and psychological changes that menopause can bring, from mood swings to anxiety and even feelings of loss and uncertainty. Together, we'll embark on an adventure to understand these changes, demystify the myths surrounding them, and empower you with strategies to not just survive but thrive during menopause.

By the end of this chapter, you will be equipped with the knowledge and tools to navigate the emotional and psychological aspects of menopause. So, let's move on this together and ensure that you emerge from it stronger, happier, and more empowered than ever before.

COPING WITH MOOD SWINGS AND EMOTIONAL TURBULENCE

Menopause can bring with it a multitude of physical changes, but the emotional and psychological shifts that often accompany this phase can be equally challenging. While each woman's experience is unique, it's essential to recognize and address the mood swings and emotional turbulence that can occur. In fact, a significant 23% of menopausal women report experiencing mood swings and emotional symptoms, according to a study by Danielle Dresden (Dresden, 2023).

Menopause is a complex transition that involves significant hormonal fluctuations. As your body adjusts to decreasing levels of estrogen and progesterone, these changes can affect your brain chemistry and, subsequently, your emotions. Several factors contribute to the mood swings experienced during menopause.

Hormonal Imbalance

The primary cause of mood swings during menopause is the hormonal imbalance. Estrogen, in particular, plays a crucial role in regulating mood and emotions. As its levels decrease, it can lead to mood swings, irritability, and increased susceptibility to stress.

Hot Flashes and Sleep Disturbances

The frequent night sweats and sleep disturbances associated with menopause can disrupt your sleep patterns. A lack of quality sleep can exacerbate mood swings and emotional instability.

Stress and Lifestyle Factors

The stress of daily life, combined with the challenges of menopause, can create a perfect storm for emotional turbulence. High stress levels and lifestyle factors like diet and exercise can influence mood swings.

Psychological Factors

The psychological impact of menopause, including concerns about aging, body image, and self-esteem, can also contribute to mood swings. This life transition often brings about feelings of uncertainty and loss, which can be emotionally challenging.

While mood swings during menopause are common, certain factors may increase your susceptibility to them. It's crucial to be aware of these potential risk factors.

Genetics

Your family history may influence your likelihood of experiencing mood swings during menopause. If your mother or grandmother went through similar emotional challenges during their menopausal years, you may be at a higher risk.

Early Menopause

Women who experience menopause at a younger age, whether naturally or due to medical intervention, may be more prone to mood swings.

Unhealthy Lifestyle

Poor diet, lack of physical activity, and smoking can all contribute to mood swings. Maintaining a healthy lifestyle can help mitigate these emotional symptoms.

Mental Health History

If you have a history of depression or anxiety, you may be at an increased risk of experiencing mood swings during menopause. It's essential to proactively manage your mental health during this time.

By understanding the causes and risk factors, you'll be better equipped to navigate these challenges and emerge from this transformative phase with fineness and strength. Remember, you are not alone, and there are solutions to help you thrive during menopause.

Mood swings during menopause can be more than just temporary emotional turbulence; they often act as a catalyst for a range of other challenges that can affect your overall well-being. Understanding the ripple effects of mood swings is vital to successfully navigating the emotional and psychological changes that accompany menopause.

DEPRESSION: A COMMON COMPANION

Depression is a condition that frequently accompanies mood swings during the menopausal transition. The hormonal imbalances and emotional fluctuations that typify this phase can trigger depressive symptoms in many women. In this setting, depression is a recognized symptom of menopause, impacting women's emotional well-being and quality of life (Dresden, 2023).

Symptoms of depression may include persistent feelings of sadness, hopelessness, and a loss of interest or pleasure in previously enjoyed activities. It can also manifest as changes in appetite, sleep disturbances, and difficulty concentrating. If you are experiencing these symptoms, it's crucial to seek help and support to manage your emotional well-being effectively.

Mood swings and depression are not the only emotional and psychological challenges that can arise during menopause. This transformative phase can bring about a variety of symptoms, including:

- Forgetfulness and brain fog: Many women report experiencing forgetfulness and difficulties with concentration during menopause. This cognitive fog can affect day-to-day functioning, causing frustration and anxiety.
- Anxiety: Anxiety, like depression, is a common symptom of menopause. Excessive worry, restlessness, and a sense of impending doom can all be part of the anxiety experience.
- Irritability and mood instability: Menopausal hormonal fluctuations can lead to irritability and

unpredictable mood swings. This can strain relationships and disrupt daily life.

- Sleep disturbances: Insomnia and night sweats can interfere with sleep, leading to exhaustion and further exacerbating mood swings and cognitive challenges.

THERAPY: A POWERFUL TOOL TO MANAGE MOOD SWINGS

One of the most effective methods for managing mood swings and the emotional and psychological challenges of menopause is therapy. Therapy can provide a safe and supportive space to explore your feelings, learn coping strategies, and develop a deeper understanding of the root causes of your emotional struggles.

Alternatively, as discussed in previous chapters, support groups can offer valuable companionship and shared experiences. Connecting with other women going through menopause can provide an additional layer of understanding and support during this life transition.

Remember, addressing these issues is a crucial step in achieving emotional well-being and thriving throughout your menopausal journey. You don't have to face these challenges alone, and there are effective tools and support systems available to help you navigate this transformative phase with empowerment.

Menopause is a phase of life marked by emotional and psychological changes, and while conventional approaches to managing these symptoms can be highly effective, it's essential to consider complementary therapies. These alternative methods can provide valuable support and contribute to a holistic approach to menopausal well-being.

St. John's Wort for Mood Swings

One complementary therapy that has gained attention for its potential to alleviate mood swings during menopause is St. John's Wort. Some research suggests that this herbal remedy may be effective in helping relieve mood swings. St. John's Wort is thought to work by influencing the levels of certain neurotransmitters in the brain, particularly serotonin, which plays a key role in regulating mood.

However, it's crucial to exercise caution when considering St. John's Wort or any other complementary therapy. This herb can interact with various medications, potentially affecting their efficacy. To ensure your safety and best results, it's advisable to discuss all your options, including complementary therapies, with a healthcare professional before incorporating them into your menopausal management plan.

Dealing With Stress

Stress is a significant contributor to mood swings and emotional turbulence during menopause. Learning to manage stress effectively can greatly improve your overall emotional and psychological well-being.

Mindfulness and Meditation

Mindfulness techniques and meditation can help you stay present in the moment and reduce anxiety. These practices teach you to manage your reactions to stressors, allowing you to respond more calmly.

- Exercise: Physical activity releases endorphins, which are natural mood lifters and can also help you sleep better, which in turn reduces stress.
- Breathing exercises: Deep breathing exercises can be done anywhere, at any time, and can quickly help you calm your nerves during a stressful moment.
- Healthy diet: A balanced diet rich in fruits, vegetables, and whole grains provides the essential nutrients your body needs to combat stress. Avoid sugar and processed foods.
- Professional help: If stress becomes overwhelming, it's wise to seek professional help from a therapist or counselor. Talking to a trained

expert can provide you with valuable coping strategies and emotional support.

Incorporating these complementary therapies and stress management techniques into your daily routine can make a significant difference in managing mood swings and emotional challenges during menopause. A well-rounded approach will ensure you thrive rather than just survive.

MINDFULNESS: AN EFFECTIVE TOOL TO REDUCE STRESS

As we navigate the emotional and psychological changes that accompany menopause, one powerful ally that can significantly improve your well-being is mindfulness. *Mindfulness* is "the practice of staying fully present in the moment, focusing on your thoughts and feelings without judgment." This approach can help you manage stress, reduce mood swings, and promote a sense of emotional balance.

When it comes to specific symptoms of menopause, mindfulness has shown promise in alleviating some of the most challenging aspects of this transition, such as hot flashes and night sweats. Research, as cited in the Balance app, has indicated that mindfulness can play a role in reducing the severity and frequency of these symptoms, potentially providing relief for women going through menopause.

Here are some simple mindfulness exercises to get you started on your path to stress reduction and emotional well-being:

- Pay attention: Mindfulness begins with being fully present in the moment. Focus on your breath, bodily sensations, or the environment around you. Pay attention to the details of your current experience.
- Practice deep breathing: One of the simplest mindfulness exercises is deep breathing. Take slow, deep breaths, paying attention to the rise and fall of your chest or the sensation of the air entering and leaving your nostrils.
- Mindfulness body scan: This exercise involves directing your attention through different parts of your body. Start at your toes and work your way up, paying attention to any tension or discomfort. This can help you release physical and emotional stress.
- Floating technique: Imagine yourself floating in a calm and peaceful body of water. As you float, let go of any tension or stress you are holding. This exercise can be a soothing way to release emotional and physical burdens.
- Gazing meditation: Find a spot to focus on, such as a candle flame or a natural scene. Gaze at it with a soft, unfocused eye. This practice can help

you calm your mind and achieve a state of mindfulness.

- Guided meditation: Utilize guided meditation sessions available online or through various apps. These sessions can provide structured guidance and can be an excellent way to incorporate mindfulness into your daily routine.

Incorporating mindfulness into your life lets you be more adept at managing the emotional and psychological changes that menopause may bring. Mindfulness enables you to reduce stress, mitigate mood swings, and regain emotional equilibrium. As you practice mindfulness, remember that it's a journey that can enhance your overall well-being and empower you to thrive during this transformative phase of life.

MANAGING ANXIETY AND DEPRESSION DURING MENOPAUSE

It's essential to address two of the most prevalent challenges: anxiety and depression. These conditions can arise from the same hormonal changes responsible for mood swings and emotional turbulence. However, understanding the impact of menopause on mental health is the first step in effectively managing these issues.

These changes can lead to:

- increased susceptibility to mood swings
- a higher likelihood of experiencing symptoms of anxiety
- a greater risk of developing depression, particularly if you have a history of mood disorders

NHS highlights how these alterations in hormone levels can affect your emotional well-being, making it essential to recognize the connection between menopause and mental health (*Menopause and Your Mental Wellbeing*, 2022).

While hormone therapy can be beneficial for addressing some menopausal symptoms, it is not a panacea for managing the psychological aspects of menopause. Namazi et al. (2019) explain that hormone therapy primarily targets physical symptoms and may not be effective for mood swings, depression, or anxiety. A holistic approach is required to address these mental health challenges.

If you're experiencing brain fog and memory issues associated with poor mental health during menopause, engaging in brain-stimulating activities can be particularly beneficial. Such activities include puzzles, memory games, and creative endeavors that challenge your cognitive abilities. These activities can help sharpen your mental faculties and make cognitive concerns less noticeable.

Here are some strategies to consider:

- Regular exercise: Engaging in regular physical activity can boost your mood and reduce feelings of anxiety and depression.
- Balanced diet: A nutritious diet rich in essential nutrients can positively impact mental health.
- Mindfulness: As discussed earlier, mindfulness practices can help alleviate stress and improve overall emotional well-being.
- Therapy: Consider therapy as a valuable resource to address and manage anxiety and depression.
- Nonhormonal medications: If necessary, discuss non-hormonal medications for depression and anxiety with your healthcare provider.

It's essential to prioritize your mental health and take proactive steps to ensure you thrive during this phase.

THERAPY OPTIONS FOR IMPROVED MENTAL HEALTH DURING MENOPAUSE

Often, managing the emotional and psychological changes that come with menopause necessitates additional support and guidance. Two effective therapeutic approaches for improving mental health during menopause are Cognitive Behavioral Therapy (CBT) and Interpersonal Therapy.

CBT is a widely recognized and highly effective approach for managing emotional and psychological challenges. It can be especially beneficial during menopause. This therapeutic method focuses on identifying negative thought patterns and behaviors and replacing them with positive ones. CBT can help you recognize and address thought patterns that contribute to mood swings, anxiety, and depression. By working with a CBT therapist, you can learn to reframe your thoughts and develop healthier coping strategies.

Interpersonal Therapy focuses on improving your relationships and communication skills. It can be particularly helpful during menopause, as this phase often brings about changes in social dynamics and relationships. This therapy can address conflicts and improve your ability to express your feelings and needs, reducing stress and emotional turbulence.

You can find suitable therapists offering CBT, Interpersonal Therapy, and other therapeutic options for menopause-related emotional and psychological issues using the Choosing Therapy directory. This tool allows you to search for therapists by location, specialization, and availability, making it easier to find a therapist who meets your specific needs.

THE GOOD NEWS: MENTAL HEALTH IMPROVES AFTER MENOPAUSE

It's important to remember that while menopause can bring emotional and psychological challenges, the good news is that mental health often improves after menopause. As explained by Waichler (2023), as hormonal fluctuations stabilize, many women experience a reduction in mood swings, anxiety, and depression. With proper support and coping strategies, you can emerge from this phase of life with enhanced emotional well-being.

In addition to therapy, you can take practical steps at home to improve your mental health and cope with emotional turmoil during menopause.

Wait With Big Decisions

Avoid making significant life decisions during this emotionally charged phase. Instead, break tasks into smaller, more manageable steps to reduce the sense of overwhelm.

Use CBT Thought Reframing

Cognitive Behavioral Therapy techniques can be applied at home. Focus on identifying negative thought patterns and replacing them with positive ones. This practice can help change the way you perceive and respond to challenges.

Cognitive Restructuring Worksheet

When necessary, use a cognitive restructuring worksheet to guide your thought-reframing process. These worksheets can help you pinpoint and reevaluate negative thought patterns and replace them with more positive and constructive ones.

By combining therapy with practical home-based techniques and a focus on self-improvement, you can effectively manage emotional and psychological changes during menopause. This comprehensive approach will empower you to thrive.

Rediscover Self-Esteem and Self-Worth During Menopause Changes

Among the aforementioned changes, it's common for women to grapple with a loss of self-esteem and self-worth. However, the good news is that you can rediscover and nurture these aspects of yourself, allowing you to thrive during menopause.

One area where women often face challenges during menopause is body image. The physical changes that accompany this phase can lead to self-esteem issues. However, it's crucial to focus on coping with these changes to improve your self-esteem. Embrace self-acceptance by accepting your body, including the changes that come with menopause. Focus on what your body can do for you rather than what it looks like. Your body is a reflection of the remarkable journey you've been on, and it's worth celebrating.

Shift your perspective from how your body looks to how it feels and functions. Prioritizing your health is an empowering way to boost self-esteem. A healthy body can help you embrace life and enjoy the activities you love.

Moreover, menopause can be an opportunity to reinvent your personal identity. Embrace the changes that come with this phase as a chance for personal growth and self-discovery. You can redefine your self-worth by exploring new interests and pursuing passions that bring you joy and fulfillment. These steps can significantly contribute to regaining and enhancing your self-esteem.

Throughout the menopausal journey, it's vital to challenge the inner critic that constantly attacks your self-worth and self-esteem. Negative self-talk can be especially damaging during this phase. Counter negative thoughts with positive affirmations, and consciously replace self-criticism with kind, supportive words. Seek support from friends, family, or a therapist about your feelings and self-esteem issues. Sharing your experiences can provide emotional support and alternative perspectives.

Consider using cognitive restructuring techniques to challenge and reframe negative thoughts that affect your self-worth. These strategies can help you combat the inner critic and nurture your self-esteem and self-worth during the changes that menopause brings.

Embracing self-acceptance, focusing on health, and challenging the inner critic are powerful tools for thriving during this phase. Your self-esteem and self-worth are valuable assets, and they deserve your care and attention as you navigate these emotional and psychological changes.

As we navigate the emotional and psychological changes during menopause, it's important to remember the wisdom of Virginia Woolf, who once said, "No need to hurry, no need to sparkle, no need to be anybody but one's self." This quote encapsulates the essence of this transformative phase in a woman's life. Menopause empowers you to be unapologetically yourself, free from societal expectations and pressures. It's a time to embrace the changes and become everything you intend to be.

With better mental health and enhanced physical wellness, you have the foundation to thrive. Now, let's shift our focus to the relationships that are integral to your well-being. By nurturing your connections with others and yourself, you can ensure that everything stays on track. Remember, your journey through menopause is not one to endure but to embrace. It's a time to be authentic, cherish your evolving self, and forge ahead with confidence and grace.

5

ESTABLISH UNSTOPPABLE RELATIONSHIPS IN MENOPAUSE

In the grand symphony of life, menopause is a unique and transformative movement, a melody of change that women across the world encounter. This chapter is a crucial note in that symphony, one that addresses a common yet often overlooked aspect of this transformative phase: the impact of menopause on our relationships.

As the curtains of menopause rise, many women find themselves facing a host of challenges, from hot flashes to mood swings, from sleep disturbances to memory lapses. These experiences are often discussed and well-documented, but there's another issue that's equally significant and far less talked about. An issue that often lurks in the shadows, quietly affecting the dynamics of our romantic relationships: low libido.

According to recent studies made by Mohsin (n.d.), a staggering 68–86.5% of women struggle with low libido during menopause. While this statistic may seem daunting, it's important to remember that it's just one facet of a multifaceted journey through menopause.

It's only one problem you face with romantic relationships. However, you need support, and that comes not just from within but also from your partner and the people around you. As you've already embarked on your journey to improve your mental health and well-being, it's essential to recognize that nurturing strong, healthy relationships is an integral part of this process.

This chapter seeks to explore the complexities of relationships during menopause and offers guidance on how to establish unstoppable connections with your loved ones. We'll delve into the various challenges you may encounter and provide strategies and insights to help you navigate these choppy waters with grace.

Menopause isn't just about hot flashes and mood swings; it's an opportunity for personal growth and transformation, a chance to revitalize your connections with those you hold dear. So, let's embark on this journey together and see what we can do to help you not only manage your moods and mental health but also build stronger, more resilient relationships that can withstand the winds of change.

NURTURING FRIENDSHIPS: THE PILLAR OF YOUR SUPPORT NETWORK

The invaluable support of friends and loved ones can make a world of difference. Building a menopause-friendly social circle to remain socially active and supported during this second coming of age is essential.

Just as our bodies undergo profound changes during menopause, our social circles also need to adapt to accommodate the evolving needs and experiences of this life phase. Building a menopause-friendly social circle is a vital first step in ensuring that your friendships continue to thrive and provide you with the support you require.

Honesty Is Key

Start by being honest with yourself. Menopause can bring about mood swings, irritability, and even moments of vulnerability. It's essential to acknowledge these changes and communicate your feelings with your friends. Understanding the shifts you're experiencing can help your friends offer support more effectively.

Adapt Social Plans and Settings

You might find that your energy levels and preferences for social activities change during menopause. Don't be afraid to alter your social plans and settings to suit everyone.

Choose activities that allow you to socialize comfortably, even when experiencing symptoms like hot flashes. Open and flexible communication with your friends is essential in ensuring that everyone feels comfortable and valued.

Don't Hesitate to Talk About Your Feelings

Menopause can be an emotionally challenging time, and it's crucial not to be afraid of talking about how you feel. Open and honest discussions with your friends about your experiences, fears, and goals can strengthen the bonds between you. Moreover, sharing your feelings can foster a deeper understanding and empathy within your social circle.

By nurturing your friendships through the ups and downs of menopause, you not only receive the emotional support you need but also create an environment where everyone feels appreciated and willing to support each other. Remember, these relationships are not just an added luxury; they're a critical part of your menopause journey. In the following sections, we'll explore more strategies for establishing and maintaining unstoppable relationships during this phase.

Strengthening Bonds Through Shared Experiences

As you embark on the path of navigating menopause and its myriad changes, one invaluable resource you can draw from is the camaraderie of friends who are in a similar phase of life. In this chapter, we explore the importance of comparing notes and swapping tips with friends who are sailing in the same boat as you. Together, we'll discover how nurturing these connections can make the menopause journey much more manageable.

Menopause is a shared experience that transcends cultural, social, and geographical boundaries. While the symptoms and challenges may vary from person to person, the underlying journey is a universal one. Remember, there's a good chance that your friends are experiencing the same emotions and issues as you during menopause. The shared camaraderie of friends who understand your struggles can be a powerful source of support and comfort.

When you can compare notes, swap tips, and maybe even share a laugh about it, you'll all find the menopause much easier to handle. Sharing your experiences and insights not only helps you gain a better understanding of your own journey but also fosters a sense of unity and empowerment among your friends. You may discover effective coping strategies, natural remedies, or even lifestyle adjustments that can alleviate the challenges of menopause.

Moreover, the act of sharing brings a certain catharsis and emotional relief. It can reduce the sense of isolation that sometimes accompanies menopause and reinforce the idea that you're not alone in this transformative journey.

By this time, you know that hormones play a significant role in our emotional and social well-being, and one hormone, in particular, stands out as crucial for nurturing relationships: progesterone. While progesterone is commonly associated with pregnancy and menstrual cycles, it also plays a vital role in maintaining and nurturing friendships throughout various phases of life, including menopause.

During menopause, hormonal imbalances can affect mood and well-being. Progesterone's role in strengthening social bonds emphasizes the importance of nurturing friendships and maintaining a support network. This hormone not only fosters emotional connection but also provides a sense of security and comfort within your relationships. Understanding the hormonal dynamics of menopause can help you appreciate the underlying reasons for mood swings and emotional fluctuations, making it easier to communicate your feelings with your friends.

In friendships, roles can shift and evolve over time. During menopause, it's essential to remember that friendships should be based on mutual support. While you may be the one experiencing menopausal symptoms, it's equally important to offer your support to friends who may be going through their unique challenges. Taking a supporting role in your friendships creates an atmosphere of reciprocity and care, ensuring that everyone feels valued.

The give-and-take of support within your social circle is a two-way street. While it's important to express your own needs and feelings, it's equally essential to be a pillar of strength and empathy for your friends. You may find that by being there for others, you create an atmosphere of trust and compassion that encourages your friends to reciprocate in kind.

Maintaining this balance is vital for the health and longevity of your friendships during menopause. When you can rely on one another for emotional support, you reinforce the bonds of your relationships, making them even more resilient in the face of life's challenges.

On the other hand, menopause can bring fluctuating energy levels, and it's essential to plan your social interactions accordingly. Be mindful of your energy peaks and valleys, and communicate them with your friends. This open and transparent approach ensures that your social interactions align with your current energy levels, allowing you to fully engage without unnecessary stress or exhaustion.

Planning your activities based on your energy levels not only benefits you but also demonstrates consideration for your friends. It allows for more enjoyable and meaningful interactions, as you can participate with enthusiasm and be fully present in the moment. In essence, it's about creating quality over quantity in your social engagements.

Through these tips, your relationships can be a source of empowerment and inspiration during this crucial phase.

THE CHANGING LANDSCAPE OF FAMILY DYNAMICS

Menopause is a journey that ripples through all aspects of our lives, including the dynamics of our closest relationships: our family. As we navigate this transformative phase, family plays a pivotal role in providing support and understanding; that's why it's important to know how family can be your greatest supporter.

Your family, whether it's your partner, children, parents, or siblings, shares a unique bond with you, and their role in your menopausal journey is immeasurable. Going through menopause can bring a myriad of emotions, physical challenges, and psychological shifts. In the midst of these changes, your family can be your greatest supporter, helping to erase feelings of isolation and offering a comforting presence during this time of transformation.

To ensure your family provides the support you need, it's essential to educate your loved ones about menopause. Menopause often remains a subject shrouded in misconceptions and stereotypes; that's why you have to get the conversation started. You can share resources, articles, and books about menopause with your family. Initiating this dialogue is the first step toward building a support system that understands your unique journey.

When your loved ones are well-informed about the physical and emotional changes associated with menopause, they can better empathize with your experiences and offer the support that aligns with your needs. As you educate them about the science and realities of menopause, you pave the way for deeper connections and smoother interactions.

Menopause symptoms may not just affect you; they can have ripple effects on your family's life as well. In this step, contemplate how your symptoms may impact your family's daily routines, dynamics, and overall well-being. Acknowledging the potential challenges that your family may face as a result of your menopausal journey is crucial. By considering these effects, you can work together to find solutions and strategies that ease the transition.

Understanding the situation from both sides—your own experiences and your family's reactions—helps in building mutual empathy and patience. It can prevent unnecessary misunderstandings and conflicts, fostering a supportive atmosphere within your family.

Open and honest communication is the linchpin of strong family relationships during menopause. Talking about your experience, you are not only letting your family know how they can support you effectively but also creating a safe space for discussing any concerns or issues that arise.

Encourage your family to ask questions and express their feelings as well. This two-way communication helps build a sense of togetherness and ensures that your family remains a pillar of strength and understanding throughout your menopausal journey.

DON'T APOLOGIZE FOR YOUR TRANSITION: MANAGING MENOPAUSAL SYMPTOMS WITH CONFIDENCE

As you navigate the transformative path of menopause, it's essential to remember one fundamental truth: You don't need to apologize for your transition. Managing the symptoms and challenges that come with this natural phase of life is an act of strength and self-empowerment. That's why we'll delve into the importance of unapologetically embracing your menopausal journey and provide guidance on managing your symptoms with confidence.

Menopause is a transition, not a setback, and certainly not something for which you should feel the need to apologize. You are not alone in this journey, and you're not the first, nor will you be the last, to experience these changes.

Own it. Don't feel shy, and do not apologize—it's just nature's way. Embrace this transition as a rite of passage, a journey that shapes you into a stronger, wiser, and more resilient woman. Your experience with menopause is a part of your life story, and it's a testament to your adaptability and endurance.

Try to explain your experience to those around you, sharing your thoughts, feelings, and the challenges you face. By opening up, you not only raise awareness about menopause but also invite understanding and empathy. Remember that by acknowledging your journey without apology, you'll emerge as a more potent force, a woman who has conquered the trials of menopause with grace and strength.

SETTING BOUNDARIES: A FOUR-STEP PROCESS

Managing your menopausal symptoms with confidence requires not only self-acceptance but also the ability to set healthy boundaries. Here's a four-step process to help you establish and maintain boundaries in your relationships and daily life:

Step 1: Self-Reflection

Begin by reflecting on your needs and priorities. What are the areas in your life where you feel the need to establish boundaries? Understand the situations and people that can trigger menopausal symptoms or emotional distress.

Step 2: Define Your Boundaries

Clearly articulate what you need to feel comfortable and supported during this transition. This might involve specifying personal space, time for self-care, or particular communication preferences. Your boundaries should be realistic and achievable.

Step 3: Communicate Your Boundaries

Share your boundaries with the people in your life, whether it's family, friends, or colleagues. Be assertive and clear in your communication. Explain the reasons behind your boundaries and how they contribute to your well-being during menopause.

Step 4: Enforce Your Boundaries

Consistently reinforce the boundaries you've set. Respectfully but firmly assert your needs, and don't feel guilty about doing so. Remember that these boundaries are essential for your physical and emotional health.

By embracing your menopausal journey without apology and setting boundaries that support your well-being, you empower yourself to manage your symptoms with confidence.

EXPLORING OPTIONS FOR INTIMACY

Menopause can bring changes to your sexual desire and function. However, there are various options and strategies to address these changes and maintain a satisfying intimate life.

Sometimes, a sexual aid can be helpful to enhance desire and pleasure. There are various products and aids available that individuals and couples may use to improve their intimate experiences.

Doctors are also studying whether a combination of estrogen and male hormones, known as androgens, may help boost sex drive in women. Discuss with your healthcare provider if this might be a suitable option for you.

Enhancing Intimacy

Intimacy is about more than just the physical act; it encompasses emotional connection and communication. Here are some strategies to enhance intimacy during menopause:

- Schedule intimate time: Make time for intimacy in your busy life. Discuss with your partner what you both enjoy and need to create a satisfying experience. Adequate rest is also crucial for maintaining physical and emotional well-being.

- Experiment more: Consider experimenting with erotic materials like videos or books, explore self-pleasure through masturbation, and introduce changes to your sexual routines to keep things exciting and fresh.
- Enjoy distraction techniques: Distraction techniques can help boost relaxation and ease anxiety, making intimacy more enjoyable. These techniques can include both erotic and nonerotic fantasies, exercises that promote relaxation and mindfulness during intimacy, and the use of music, videos, or television to set the mood.
- Variety is the spice of life: Keep your intimate life vibrant by introducing variety. Experiment with different settings, positions, and forms of physical and emotional connection.

Intimacy is a multifaceted gem that can bring you and your partner closer, increase your desire, and reinforce the bonds that make your relationship unstoppable. While physical intimacy is often the first that comes to mind, other vital forms of intimacy matter greatly.

Physical Intimacy

Physical intimacy includes gestures like holding hands, hugs, kisses, and cuddling. Affectionate touch is closely related to the emotional connection between partners, nurturing closeness and a sense of security.

Emotional Intimacy

Emotional intimacy is about "sharing your feelings, thoughts, and experiences with your partner. It's the sense of being emotionally close and connected, understanding each other deeply, and feeling safe to express vulnerabilities."

Intellectual Intimacy

Intellectual intimacy revolves around "sharing ideas, engaging in meaningful conversations, and being open to different perspectives. It fosters mental connection and stimulates the growth of the relationship through intellectual stimulation."

Spiritual Intimacy

Spiritual intimacy pertains to "shared beliefs, values, and the quest for meaning and purpose in life. It's about finding connection and harmony in your spiritual or philosophical viewpoints and deepening your bond through shared values and aspirations."

Social Intimacy

Social intimacy involves "engaging in social activities together, building a strong social support system, and having shared social circles." It's about finding compatibility in the way you connect with friends, family, and the outside world, creating a fulfilling social life as a couple.

During menopause, exploring these various forms of intimacy can help maintain and strengthen the bond with your partner. It's not just about physical closeness; it's about nurturing all aspects of your connection, ensuring that your relationship remains vibrant, resilient, and deeply connected.

CONTRACEPTION IN MENOPAUSE

Contraception during menopause is a relevant and sometimes overlooked topic. The need for contraception largely depends on your individual circumstances. Menopause is considered to be complete when you haven't had a period for a year or when your healthcare provider confirms that you've reached menopause. However, it's crucial to note that menopause can be confirmed only in retrospect, and the months leading up to it—perimenopause—can still be fertile.

If you're sexually active and don't wish to become pregnant, it's essential to use contraception until menopause is confirmed. Some women also choose to continue using contraception for noncontraceptive reasons, such as regulating menstrual cycles, managing symptoms, or preventing certain medical conditions.

Discuss your specific needs and concerns with your healthcare provider to determine the most suitable contraceptive options for you during menopause. It's a personal decision that should align with your individual health and lifestyle. Remember that open communication with your partner and healthcare provider can guide you in making the right choices for your sexual health during this transformative phase of life.

J. K. Rowling, the celebrated author of the Harry Potter series, aptly noted, "Family is a lifejacket in the stormy sea of life." This quote beautifully encapsulates the pivotal role of our loved ones during turbulent times of change.

Keeping your family, partner, and friends close for support is not just a choice; it's a lifeline that will help you embrace the transition more smoothly, even in the seemingly stormy waters of menopause. In the chapters ahead, we'll delve deeper into how to strengthen these invaluable relationships and, in turn, find the balance between your personal and professional life.

In the face of the challenges that menopause may bring, the bonds you've nurtured and the support you've cultivated will serve as your anchors, steadying you as you navigate the winds of change. In the next chapter, let's set sail and explore how to maintain harmony in your work-life balance during this transformative phase.

INTERACTIVE ELEMENT: THE INTIMACY CHALLENGE

Building and maintaining intimacy in your relationships is an essential aspect of navigating menopause with grace. To help you strengthen your bonds and enhance all facets of intimacy, I challenge you to embark on an Intimacy Challenge.

Challenge: For the next few weeks, aim to engage in an intimacy-building activity with your partner every second or third night. The goal is to focus on improving each level of intimacy—physical, emotional, intellectual, spiritual, and social. Here's how you can get started:

- Physical intimacy: Start with gestures of physical affection. Try holding hands, hugging, kissing, or cuddling before sleep. These small acts of physical closeness can set the stage for a more profound connection.
- Emotional intimacy: Dedicate time to deep conversations about your feelings, experiences, and dreams. Share your vulnerabilities and allow your partner to do the same. By opening up emotionally, you'll strengthen your emotional connection.
- Intellectual intimacy: Engage in discussions about topics that interest both of you. Share your thoughts on books, movies, or current events.

Intellectual intimacy can be as simple as exchanging ideas and perspectives.

- Spiritual intimacy: Explore your spiritual beliefs and values together. Discuss how your beliefs align and where they differ. This shared exploration can deepen your spiritual connection.
- Social intimacy: Plan activities that you both enjoy with your social circle, whether it's spending time with friends, attending events, or participating in hobbies together. Strengthening your social bonds can be a fun and enriching experience.

Set a schedule that works for both you and your partner, whether it's every second or third night, and commit to this challenge. As you embark on this journey, you'll find that the process of actively nurturing your various levels of intimacy can bring you and your partner closer and help you embrace the changes of menopause.

Feel free to share your experiences, progress, and any insights you gain during this challenge with fellow readers in the community. Together, we can empower each other to build unstoppable relationships during menopause.

6

CREATE THE IDEAL WORK-LIFE BALANCE AND SAFEGUARD FUTURE PLANS

Now, we start a crucial chapter that centers on the delicate balance between personal and professional goals during the transformative phase of menopause. This chapter sheds light on the profound impact that menopause can have on our work life and how safeguarding our future plans becomes essential.

Picture this: You've reached a point in life where you are discovering new facets of yourself, embracing the wisdom that comes with age, and stepping into a future full of promise. Menopause is a unique juncture in a woman's life, marked by both challenges and opportunities, but it should never deter you from pursuing your dreams and aspirations.

Now, let me share a startling statistic with you: A remarkable 40% of women report that menopause affects their work performance and productivity on a weekly basis

(Castrillon, 2023). This, indeed, is a concerning revelation. Struggling at work due to the symptoms and changes that menopause brings can significantly undermine the progress you've made on your MENO-WISE journey toward a happier, healthier life.

However, this chapter is here to guide you toward a solution. In the coming pages, we will explore strategies and insights to help you create the ideal work-life balance and secure your future plans. The aim is to ensure that both your personal and professional life not only remain intact but thrive during this transformative phase. We will empower you with the knowledge and tools you need to navigate this remarkable chapter of your life with dignity and trust.

Understanding that menopause should not be a roadblock but a stepping stone to a more empowered and fulfilled future, let's work toward a harmonious blend of personal and professional aspirations, ensuring that nothing stands in the way of your MENO-WISE success.

Menopause is a significant life transition that can sometimes bring unexpected challenges, particularly in the workplace. It's crucial to acknowledge these challenges and find constructive ways to address them. Open and effective communication is key to navigating this phase and ensuring that your professional life remains as fulfilling as ever.

One of the first and most vital steps in managing work-related challenges during menopause is to engage in open and honest conversations with your employers. It's essential to foster a workplace environment that is not only inclusive but also considerate of the unique needs and experiences of women going through menopause.

Studies and articles like the one by Caroline Castrillon on Forbes titled "Why It's Time to Address Menopause in the Workplace" highlight the importance of addressing menopause-related issues in the professional sphere. The most powerful changes often happen when these discussions take place in the boardroom, leading to more inclusive and supportive workplace policies and practices.

TALK TO YOUR EMPLOYER: THE FIRST STEP TOWARD FLEXIBILITY

Initiating a conversation with your employer is often the first step in seeking the flexibility and accommodations you may require during menopause. This dialogue can be a pivotal moment in ensuring that both you and your workplace are in sync with your unique needs.

The Hello Magazine article titled "Flexible Work: What Menopausal Women Need to Know" provides valuable insights into how you can make the most of these discussions. The article suggests that your first step should be to talk to your employer. Thus, express your interest in exploring flexible working arrangements and accommodations that can support you effectively.

Explaining How Menopause Affects Your Work

To gain your employer's understanding and support for flexible working arrangements, it is essential to communicate how menopause affects your work and why these changes are necessary. By helping your manager comprehend the impact of menopause on your work life, you create an environment of empathy and cooperation that can be beneficial for both parties. Here are five steps to guide you in this process to effectively speak to your employer about menopause:

Step 1: Choose the Right Time and Place—Schedule a Meeting

Select a suitable time and place to have this conversation. Ideally, it should be a private and relaxed setting where both you and your employer can focus without distractions.

Step 2: Research and Prepare for the Discussion

Before the conversation, prepare a brief but comprehensive overview of how menopause is affecting your work. List the specific symptoms or challenges you are facing and how they impact your productivity and well-being.

Research the relevant company policies regarding health and wellness. Be prepared with facts and figures about how menopause can affect productivity. The Forbes article mentioned earlier provides valuable insights to support your case.

Step 3: Be Open and Honest and Share Your Goals

During the conversation, be candid about your experiences with menopause and how it may affect your work. Share your concerns and challenges honestly, emphasizing that you are seeking a solution to maintain your performance. Express your commitment to your role and your desire to continue performing at your best. Emphasize your long-term dedication to the company and your role in its success.

Step 4: Suggest Solutions

It's helpful to come to the discussion with potential solutions or accommodations that could make your work environment more supportive during this transition. This proactive approach demonstrates your commitment to finding mutually beneficial solutions. For example, flexible work hours, remote work options, or adjustments to your workload during particularly challenging times.

Step 5: Seek Mutual Agreement by Highlighting Mutual Benefits

Engage in a constructive dialogue with your employer, aiming for a mutually agreed-upon plan that considers both your needs and the requirements of the job. Encourage ongoing communication to ensure the plan is effective and adaptable.

By initiating this open dialogue, you not only advocate for your own well-being but also contribute to a broader cultural shift in how menopause is perceived and accommodated in the workplace. The power of these conversations lies not only in the improvements they can bring to your personal work experience but also in the positive impact they can have on the lives of countless other women who may follow in your footsteps.

Remember, menopause is not a challenge to overcome; it is a transformative journey that, when managed effectively, can become a source of empowerment and growth.

In our journey through the transformative phase of menopause, one of the most valuable tools at our disposal is the concept of flexibility. Navigating the challenges of menopause while maintaining a thriving career is made considerably more manageable through the exploration of flexible work arrangements and accommodations.

Explain how these accommodations can benefit both you and the organization. Emphasize that a healthier and happier workforce can lead to increased productivity and reduced absenteeism.

By proactively addressing the impact of menopause on your work life and proposing thoughtful solutions, you not only create an atmosphere of collaboration but also increase the likelihood of securing the flexibility and accommodations you need. This dialogue can lead to a win-win situation, where your professional life remains intact and thriving, and your employer benefits from a more content and productive workforce.

With open communication and understanding, we can ensure that it becomes a stepping stone to greater empowerment and success.

In the next sections of this chapter, we'll delve deeper into strategies for maintaining a healthy work-life balance and securing your future plans during menopause, ensuring that this phase becomes a catalyst for your continued success.

ADJUSTMENTS FOR PERSONAL AND PROFESSIONAL GOALS

Menopause is a unique journey, and as we navigate its challenges, we need to consider adjustments that align with our professional and personal aspirations. Flexibility and accommodations can be the key to maintaining your work-life balance while safeguarding your future plans.

When it comes to making adjustments during menopause, it's essential to tailor them to your specific needs, taking into account both your personal and professional goals. Not every woman's experience with menopause is the same, so what works for one may not work for another. Here are some potential adjustments to consider:

- Flexible work hours: Adjusting your work hours to accommodate your energy levels and symptom management. This may involve starting and ending your workday at different times to suit your needs. Requesting adjusted start and end times or compressed workweeks can provide you with more control over your schedule.
- Remote work options: Exploring the possibility of working from home or telecommuting, which can be especially beneficial during days when symptoms are particularly challenging.
- Reduced workload: Discussing the potential to reduce your workload or responsibilities temporarily to allow for better self-care and symptom management.
- Leave policies: Understanding your company's leave policies and considering whether intermittent leaves or additional sick days might be necessary during severe symptoms.
- Adjusted breaks: Incorporating more frequent, shorter breaks into your workday to manage hot flashes, fatigue, or other symptoms effectively.

- Job sharing: Exploring job-sharing arrangements with a colleague can help distribute workload and responsibilities while providing you with essential support.

Everyone experiences perimenopause and menopause differently, so it's important to work with your employer to find the best solutions for your unique situation.

REDEFINING PERSONAL AND PROFESSIONAL GOALS FOR BALANCE

Embracing the transformation and striving for the ideal work-life balance often requires us to reevaluate our personal and professional goals. This realignment can serve as a compass to navigate the discussions around flexible working arrangements with your manager or employer while also ensuring you find excitement and fulfillment outside of work.

Before you redefine your goals, it's crucial to recognize the need for balance in both your work and personal life. Menopause can bring about physical and emotional changes that necessitate adjustments in various aspects of life.

Reevaluating Professional Goals

As you navigate the world of work, it's essential to consider how menopause may influence your professional goals. Here are some steps to consider:

Align Career Goals With Personal Well-being

Assess your current career goals and determine if they align with your well-being during menopause. If your current trajectory is causing excessive stress, consider reshaping your goals to prioritize your health and comfort.

Explore Opportunities for Flexible Work Arrangements

If you find that the demands of your current role are challenging to manage, explore opportunities for flexible work hours or remote work. Redefining your professional goals may involve a discussion with your employer to adjust your work arrangements accordingly.

Seek Opportunities for Growth and Learning

This phase of life presents an opportunity to explore new career avenues or seek additional training that aligns with your interests and health needs. Don't be afraid to pivot or consider new possibilities.

Reimagine Personal Goals

Beyond your career, it's equally essential to set personal goals that balance the excitement and responsibilities outside work. Here are some steps to guide you:

- Prioritize self-care: Set personal goals that prioritize your health and well-being. This may include adopting a regular exercise routine, maintaining a balanced diet, or incorporating relaxation techniques into your daily life.
- Cultivate hobbies and interests: Rediscover or develop hobbies and interests that bring you joy and relaxation outside work. These activities can provide a refreshing break from the daily routine.
- Embrace new opportunities: The Balance Menopause article titled "How to Set Goals to Boost Your Health and Happiness" encourages embracing new opportunities. Don't be afraid to try new things, explore new passions, or embark on adventures you've always dreamt of but never had the time for.

Redefining your personal and professional goals, you are ensuring that your work-life balance is well-maintained, allowing you to address the changes that come with menopause while continuing to pursue a fulfilling life. Don't hesitate to seek support and guidance as you realign your goals, and remember that this is a transformative period that can lead to newfound empowerment and happiness.

PURSUING PASSIONS AND HOBBIES FOR BALANCE AND MOTIVATION

Finding and pursuing passions and hobbies are essential components of creating the ideal work-life balance and safeguarding our future plans. These interests not only guide our goals and motivation in both professional and personal life but also serve as a source of joy and fulfillment. Let's explore how you can harness your passions and hobbies to find balance and motivation.

Consider What You Already Enjoy

One of the first steps in pursuing passions and hobbies is to consider what you already enjoy. Think about the activities that make you lose track of time and leave you feeling invigorated. Reflecting on what you enjoy can lead you to activities that fuel your enthusiasm.

Explore Connections

Passions and hobbies can often be discovered by exploring connections between seemingly unrelated interests. These intersections can spark new passions and provide fresh perspectives. When you look for the common threads among your interests, you might find a unique passion at the intersection of these ingredients.

Distinguish Hobbies from Profitable Passions

While hobbies are enjoyable activities, some passions can also translate into profitable ventures. Distinguishing between the two is essential. What may feel like play can become a potential source of income or a fulfilling side project. In your pursuit of passions, don't be afraid to explore how these interests can be integrated into your professional life.

Challenge Fears and Find Your Next Step

Discovering and pursuing passions and hobbies can be an exciting yet challenging journey. Fear of the unknown or doubts about your abilities may hold you back. However, it's vital to challenge these fears and take the next step. The act of exploration itself can be incredibly motivating and fulfilling. Whether it's taking a class, attending a workshop, or simply dedicating time to your chosen interest, each step you take brings you closer to realizing your passions.

In the context of menopause, finding and nurturing these passions and hobbies can be particularly empowering. They provide an outlet for self-expression, stress relief, and personal growth, contributing to a well-rounded and balanced life. Whether you're seeking motivation at work, looking to explore new opportunities, or simply aiming to enjoy your personal life to the fullest, your passions and hobbies can guide you.

SETTING GOALS TO GUIDE YOUR CHOICES DURING MENOPAUSE

Setting clear and meaningful goals is a fundamental aspect of navigating the transformative journey of menopause with grace. These goals serve as a roadmap, guiding your choices and actions in both your professional and personal life.

Define Your Goals Thoroughly

Define your goals comprehensively, taking into account both your work and personal life. "The Balance Menopause" article on setting goals emphasizes the importance of clarity when defining your goals. Knowing what you want and why you want it is the first step toward success.

Adopt the Do Approach

Plan to *do* rather than just *be*. In other words, set specific and actionable goals. Instead of saying, "I'll be healthier," say, "I'll exercise for 30 minutes 3 times a week." The *do approach* makes your goals more actionable and easier to measure, ensuring that you have a clear path.

Aim for Growth Goals

Make sure your goals focus on growth, both personal and professional. Setting goals that encourage growth can be particularly empowering during menopause, as this phase offers a unique opportunity for self-discovery and development. Aim to grow in areas that matter most to you and align with your overall well-being.

Choose Goals That Motivate You

Select goals that genuinely motivate you. Your goals should be driven by passion and desire, as motivation plays a significant role in your ability to follow through. When you're passionate about your goals, you're more likely to stay committed and enthusiastic about achieving them.

Design Action and Coping Plans

To ensure the success of your goals, design action and coping plans that match them. These plans outline the specific steps you need to take to achieve your goals, as well as strategies for coping with any challenges or setbacks that may arise along the way. Having these plans in place increases your chances of reaching your objectives.

Following these steps and setting clear, meaningful goals, you can navigate menopause with a sense of purpose and direction. These goals will guide your choices in both your professional and personal life, helping you maintain a healthy work-life balance while safeguarding your future plans. In the subsequent sections of this chapter, we'll go deeper into strategies for embracing new opportunities and securing your future during this remarkable journey of change and empowerment.

FINANCIAL PLANNING AND RETIREMENT CONSIDERATIONS FOR THE SECOND COMING OF AGE

As you embrace the transformative phase of menopause, it's essential to consider the financial aspects of this journey. Menopause can impact your financial well-being, and with careful planning and consideration, you can safeguard your retirement and ensure a financially secure future.

Menopause can have financial implications for retirement, contributing to the gender retirement gap. Remember that menopause is not just a health issue; it's a financial one as well. Women experiencing severe menopausal symptoms may take time off work, work part-time, or even leave their jobs prematurely, affecting their retirement savings.

To bridge the menopause retirement gap, professional financial advice can be invaluable. Expert advice helps you make informed decisions about your retirement planning. Financial advisors assist in designing a retirement plan that accounts for any potential disruptions due to menopause and ensures you can achieve the retirement lifestyle you desire.

If you have a 401(k) or other retirement plans, it's essential to periodically check them to assess your savings. Review your contributions, investment choices, and retirement goals. Make necessary adjustments to align your retirement plans with your evolving financial needs, especially considering the potential impact of menopause.

Reassess your lifestyle and spending habits. Determine whether there are areas where you can cut costs or reallocate funds to boost your retirement savings. Be mindful of your financial priorities, especially when faced with the additional financial challenges that may accompany menopause.

On the other hand, explore diversified investment options to secure your financial future. Investing in assets like the housing market can provide alternative avenues for growing your wealth. Diversification may help mitigate risks and provide financial stability, particularly during life's transitions.

Lastly, it's crucial to regularly review and monitor your retirement plan, savings, and overall financial state. Even if you choose to do this with the help of a financial expert, staying informed and proactive about your finances is essential for ensuring that your retirement remains on track.

Navigating the financial implications of menopause and retirement planning requires diligence and consideration. By addressing these financial aspects and seeking expert guidance when necessary, you can safeguard your future and embark on this transformative journey with confidence.

Oprah Winfrey once wisely noted, "I've learned that you can't have everything and do everything at the same time." Her words resonate deeply with the core theme of this chapter, where we explore the delicate art of balancing work, personal life, and financial planning during menopause. The journey through menopause is a transformative one, requiring us to make conscious choices and prioritize what matters most.

As we gracefully enter the golden years, it becomes clear that we must focus on each aspect of our lives with intention and purpose. Whether it's our careers, personal aspirations, or financial well-being, careful planning is the key to ensuring that menopause doesn't debilitate us but rather empowers us to navigate this phase of life with classiness.

This chapter has taken us through strategies to create the ideal work-life balance, safeguard our financial future, and set meaningful goals. It's a journey that requires a holistic approach, one that extends beyond traditional methods. In the next section, we'll delve into holistic and alternative methods to manage menopause because embracing change and thriving through this transition is not solely about work and finances; it's also about nurturing our well-being and celebrating the beauty of each passing day.

INTERACTIVE ELEMENT: DAILY MOOD CHART FOR EMBRACING CHANGE

As you journey through the transformative phase of menopause and explore new career paths, passions, and hobbies, it's crucial to stay attuned to your emotions and well-being. To help you record and analyze how your moods change, consider using the daily mood chart below. This simple tool can provide valuable insights into the emotional impact of your choices and activities as you embrace change and empower yourself. By tracking your daily moods, you can gain a better understanding of how embracing new career paths, passions, and hobbies impacts your well-being. This self-awareness can help you make informed choices that align with your emotional needs and empower you to address the challenges and opportunities of menopause.

Instructions

- Date: Write the date at the top of each column.
- Mood: In the *Mood* column, rate your mood on a scale from 1–10, with 1 being the lowest—terrible—and 10 the highest—excellent.
- Morning: Record your mood in the morning, right after waking up. How do you feel as you start your day?
- Midday: In the middle of the day, assess your mood. Has it changed? Why has it changed?
- Evening: Before bedtime, reflect on how your mood has evolved throughout the day. Note any specific events or activities that influenced your emotions.

Tips

- Be honest and consistent when rating your mood.
- Identify patterns or triggers that affect your mood. Is there a correlation between certain activities and your emotional state?
- Use this chart as a tool for self-reflection and personal growth.
- Adjust the chart to suit your specific needs and preferences.

7

PICK HOLISTIC METHODS TO MASTER MENOPAUSE DAILY

Welcome to the heart of your journey, where we delve into holistic approaches to master menopause. Just as we've navigated mental health and physical symptoms in previous chapters, this section will empower you with alternative methods that can help you embrace this transformative phase.

Menopause, often referred to as the *second coming of age*, can be a challenging transition for many women. It brings a myriad of physical, emotional, and psychological changes that can impact your daily life. But, here's the exciting news: Over 50% of women have discovered the power of complementary and alternative medicine in managing menopause's long-term effects. (Posadzki et al., 2013).

In this chapter, we will explore holistic methods, complementary medicine, and the wonders of natural superfoods to help you navigate the unique challenges menopause presents. These methods are designed to empower you to take control of your journey, minimize discomfort, and enhance your overall well-being as you transition into this phase.

Are you ready to discover the transformative potential of holistic approaches and alternative therapies to master menopause daily? Let's move on this empowering journey together and show you how to face the second coming of age.

YOGA: A HOLISTIC APPROACH TO MANAGING MENOPAUSE

In the journey of menopause, embracing holistic methods can be a game-changer, offering benefits that go beyond merely maintaining strength, healthier bones, and sustainable muscle mass. One such holistic practice gaining recognition for its incredible advantages is yoga. The ancient practice of yoga encompasses more than just physical exercise; it also encloses controlled breathing and meditation, creating a mind-body connection that can help you master menopause.

Yoga has been praised for its numerous health benefits, and it plays a significant role in managing the challenges of menopause. Controlled breathing and yoga stretches, also known as asanas, can work wonders for women going through this transformative phase.

The Magic of Yoga in Menopause

Studies have shown that yoga can be a powerful tool in managing menopausal symptoms. It promotes emotional well-being and has a calming effect on the mind. In addition, yoga can help alleviate hot flashes, mood swings, and the discomfort of cramps, all of which are common symptoms during menopause. Furthermore, this ancient practice has been found to reduce stress, anxiety, and insomnia, making it an invaluable asset for women navigating this transition.

But it's not just about the physical and emotional benefits; yoga offers a social aspect as well. Joining a local yoga class specifically designed for women experiencing menopause can be a source of camaraderie and support. Sharing this journey with other women who understand what you're going through can provide a significant boost to your emotional well-being, making the path through menopause a bit smoother.

Popular Yoga Poses for Menopause

Now, you might be wondering which yoga poses are particularly beneficial during menopause. Here are some that have earned praise for their potential to provide relief from various menopausal symptoms:

- Butterfly pose: Ideal for indigestion, this pose can help ease digestive discomfort and promote relaxation.
- Reclining bound angle pose: This pose is beneficial for headaches, insomnia, irritability, and anxiety. It helps you find calmness and balance.
- Garland pose: Known for stress reduction and an energy boost, the garland pose can help you maintain your vitality.
- Forward bent pose: Excellent for addressing cramps, heart palpitations, mood swings, and hot flashes, this pose improves blood flow, prevents cramps, and stabilizes the heart rate.
- Cobra pose: If you're looking to manage weight, indigestion, or insomnia, the cobra pose can help you achieve your goals. Regular practice can relieve stress and anxiety, induce a sense of calmness, and contribute to a good night's sleep.

As you explore the benefits of yoga during menopause, remember that consistency is key. Incorporating these poses into your daily routine can contribute to your overall well-being during this phase of life. By embracing the holistic practice of yoga, you can empower yourself to manage menopause, enhancing your physical and emotional resilience throughout this journey.

MEDITATION: A MINDFUL APPROACH TO EMBRACING MENOPAUSE

In the journey through menopause, embracing holistic methods is crucial, and among them, meditation stands out as a powerful tool. While mindfulness meditation is already known for its stress-reducing benefits, what many women may not be aware of is that specific meditation styles can be tailored to target and alleviate the symptoms associated with menopause.

Meditation is an excellent tool to help women navigate the transformative phase of menopause. Its primary strength lies in its ability to cultivate mindfulness, fostering a deeper connection between the mind and body. By practicing meditation regularly, you can enhance your emotional well-being, reduce stress, and develop a heightened awareness of your body's changes during this time.

The meditation styles adapted to address the unique challenges of menopause can provide targeted relief from symptoms like hot flashes, mood swings, and anxiety, making them invaluable additions to your menopause empowerment toolkit.

Here are some meditation techniques that can target particular menopausal challenges, offering you relief and empowerment in the process.

Sensory Meditation for Anxiety Relief

Menopause often brings a wave of anxiety, and sensory meditation can be your guiding light in calming the mind and finding serenity. This technique focuses on engaging your senses to bring your attention to the present moment. By honing in on your sensory experiences—what you see, hear, touch, taste, and smell—you can redirect your thoughts away from anxious ruminations.

Sensory meditation invites you to immerse yourself in the sensory richness of the world around you, making it challenging for anxiety to take center stage. This technique can provide a powerful sense of relaxation and tranquility, allowing you to navigate anxiety with confidence.

Loving-Kindness Meditation for Self-Esteem and Emotional Well-Being

Menopause often comes with a range of emotions, including self-esteem issues and emotional turmoil linked to changes in your body image. Loving-kindness meditation, also known as *Metta*, can be a powerful practice to enhance self-compassion and emotional resilience during this time.

Loving-kindness meditation encourages you to cultivate feelings of love, compassion, and kindness, first toward yourself and then toward others. By fostering self-love and self-acceptance, you can ease the emotional burden that may arise due to the physical changes menopause brings. This meditation practice empowers you to embrace your evolving self, celebrating your inner strength and beauty.

Bedtime Meditation for Improved Sleep

One of the most common challenges during menopause is disrupted sleep. Many women find it difficult to achieve restful, rejuvenating sleep, which can lead to daytime fatigue and irritability. Bedtime meditation is a tailored solution to help you unwind and improve your sleep quality.

This meditation practice involves relaxation techniques and guided visualizations specifically designed to prepare your mind and body for a peaceful night's sleep. By calming your thoughts and easing physical tension, bedtime meditation can help you overcome sleep disturbances, ensuring you wake up refreshed and ready to face each day with vitality.

By incorporating these targeted meditation techniques into your daily routine, you can address the specific challenges that menopause brings, whether it's anxiety, self-esteem issues, or sleep disturbances. Each meditation style empowers you to navigate menopause with grace, resilience, and a deep sense of self-awareness.

ACUPUNCTURE: A HOLISTIC APPROACH TO LONG-TERM MENOPAUSE SYMPTOM RELIEF

In the quest to master menopause, we explore various holistic methods, each offering a unique pathway to empower women during this transformative phase. Among these holistic approaches, acupuncture emerges as a powerful tool that can provide long-term relief from menopausal symptoms, offering a holistic approach to managing the changes that come with this stage of life.

Acupuncture, an ancient healing practice rooted in Traditional Chinese Medicine (TCM), has been used for centuries to treat a wide range of health issues, including those associated with menopause. It involves the insertion of fine, sterile needles at specific points on the body, known as acupuncture points, to stimulate energy flow or qi.

But how does acupuncture work to alleviate menopausal symptoms? The magic of acupuncture lies in its ability to balance the body's vital energy, which can become disrupted during menopause. Targeting specific acupuncture points, practitioners aim to restore harmony within the body, promoting physical and emotional well-being.

One of the remarkable aspects of acupuncture is its ability to provide fast and effective relief from menopausal symptoms. Many women find that after just a few sessions, they experience significant improvements in their overall well-being. Here's how acupuncture can help:

Hot Flashes and Night Sweats

Acupuncture has been shown to reduce the frequency and severity of hot flashes and night sweats. By targeting specific points, it can regulate the body's temperature control mechanisms, providing relief from these often distressing symptoms.

Mood Swings and Anxiety

Acupuncture can have a calming effect on the nervous system, helping to alleviate mood swings and anxiety. It promotes the release of endorphins, the body's natural feel-good chemicals, which can ease emotional turbulence.

Sleep Disturbances

Many women experience sleep disturbances during menopause, and acupuncture can help improve sleep quality by promoting relaxation and reducing the factors that disrupt restful sleep.

Hormone Regulation

Acupuncture may assist in regulating hormonal fluctuations during menopause, which can contribute to symptom relief.

The beauty of acupuncture as a holistic approach to managing menopause is that it treats the whole person, addressing the physical, emotional, and energetic aspects of this life stage. With acupuncture, you can find long-term relief from the challenges of menopause, enabling you to navigate this transition with greater ease and resilience.

So, whether you're seeking fast relief from troublesome symptoms or a comprehensive approach to managing menopause, acupuncture can be a valuable addition to your menopause empowerment toolkit. It offers a holistic pathway to help you embrace the changes and uncertainties of this phase of life, allowing you to move forward with vitality.

HERBAL REMEDIES AND NATURAL SUPPLEMENTS: HARNESSING HOLISTIC SOLUTIONS FOR MENOPAUSE

It's essential to explore holistic approaches that can help alleviate the wide range of symptoms that accompany this transformative phase of life. Herbal remedies and natural supplements are among the options that have gained attention for their potential to make menopausal symptoms feel less intense. However, it's crucial to approach these remedies with caution, as their efficacy can vary, and they may interact with prescription medications. Let's explore some of the best-known herbal remedies and natural supplements for managing menopause:

Black Cohosh

Black cohosh has garnered scientific attention for its potential to relieve menopausal symptoms such as hot flashes. It is believed to influence estrogen receptors in the body, which may help mitigate some symptoms.

Red Clover

Red clover is another herbal remedy that has been explored for its potential to alleviate hot flashes and other menopausal symptoms. It contains compounds called isoflavones, which may have a mild estrogen-like effect.

Dong Quai

Dong Quai, often referred to as *female ginseng*, is an herb that is sometimes used to relieve menopausal symptoms. However, it should be used with caution, especially if you have uterine fibroids.

Kava

Kava is known for its calming effects and is sometimes used to address anxiety and mood swings during menopause. However, it's essential to be cautious with kava, as it may have potential safety concerns and may be regulated in some regions.

Korean Ginseng

Korean ginseng is a popular adaptogenic herb that may promote overall well-being, reduce stress, and improve energy levels during menopause.

Horny Goat Weed

Horny goat weed has traditionally been used for sexual health and may have some potential benefits during menopause. Nevertheless, it's important to note that there are no clinical studies supporting its effectiveness.

Hops

Hops, the female flowers of the hop plant, contain a potent phytoestrogen known as 8-prenylnaringenin, which may offer some relief from hot flashes.

St. John's Wort

While St. John's Wort is often associated with mood support, it may have potential benefits for managing menopausal mood swings and emotional fluctuations.

Valerian and Soy Isoflavones

Valerian is known for its calming and sleep-promoting effects, which can be valuable for women experiencing sleep disturbances during menopause. Soy isoflavones, which mimic estrogen in the body, have shown promise in managing menopausal symptoms.

As with any natural remedies, it's crucial to consult with a healthcare professional before incorporating these herbal remedies and supplements into your menopause management plan. They can provide guidance on the safety and potential interactions with other medications you may be taking. With proper care and caution, herbal remedies and natural supplements can be valuable additions to your holistic approach to mastering menopause.

THE ROLE OF SUPERFOODS IN LONG-TERM MENOPAUSE SYMPTOM MANAGEMENT

When it comes to navigating the intricate landscape of menopause, nutrition plays a vital role. You might have heard about the importance of a balanced diet in managing immediate menopausal symptoms, but there are a few hidden gems, secret superfoods, that can significantly contribute to symptom management over the years. These superfoods aren't often discussed, but they have the potential to make your menopause journey more comfortable and empowering.

Flaxseed

Flaxseed is a nutritional powerhouse. Its high fiber content helps manage digestive issues that sometimes accompany menopause. It's also rich in lignans, which may provide relief from hot flashes.

Leafy Greens

Fill your plate with leafy greens such as kale, spinach, and Swiss chard. These vegetables are packed with essential nutrients like calcium and vitamin K, which support bone health and help maintain strong bones during menopause.

Cold Water Fish

Fish are very rich in omega-3. You can eat sardines, tuna, salmon, the one you like. These healthy fats help reduce inflammation, support cardiovascular health, and contribute to overall well-being during menopause.

Prunes

Estrogen deficiency during menopause can lead to digestive issues. Prunes are a natural remedy that helps maintain healthy digestion and alleviate constipation.

Dark Chocolate

Dark chocolate is a delightful treat that can provide mood-boosting benefits. It contains compounds that may help improve mood and reduce emotional fluctuations, which are common during menopause.

Kimchi

Kimchi is a fermented food that belongs to the superfood category due to its probiotic content. Probiotics can support gut health, which is closely linked to overall well-being. Other fermented foods like kefir and sauerkraut are also valuable additions to your diet.

Maca

Maca is a root vegetable known for its potential to alleviate menopausal symptoms. It may help reduce hot flashes, improve mood, and boost overall energy levels.

By incorporating these superfoods into your diet, you can proactively manage menopausal symptoms over the years, promoting a smoother and more comfortable transition. Keep in mind that while these superfoods can offer valuable benefits, a balanced diet with a variety of nutrient-rich foods is key to comprehensive menopause management. So, let's embrace these secret superfoods as your allies on this empowering journey through menopause.

Robert Urich said, "A healthy outside starts from the inside." As we journey through the pages of this book, these words resonate deeply with our mission. We've embarked on a path of holistic and complementary treatments, embracing management tools that not only help us weather the challenges of menopause but also ensure lasting joy and wellness, both during and after this transformative phase.

The MENO-WISE journey has been a comprehensive exploration of various strategies and techniques, empowering you to navigate menopause with grace. We've delved into mental health, physical well-being, holistic remedies, and nutrition, all aimed at equipping you with the tools to thrive during this significant life transition.

And now, as we stand on the threshold of the final step in our MENO-WISE journey, let's contemplate the idea of lasting, for the choices you make today, the wisdom you've gathered, and the empowerment you've embraced will continue to resonate throughout your life's chapters.

The next step will guide you in gracefully embracing the years to come. It will be a celebration of wisdom, strength, and beauty, ensuring that you continue to lead a life filled with vitality, resilience, and joy. As we transition into this last phase of our journey, remember that the empowering tools you've collected thus far will serve as the foundation for this future exploration.

So, let's continue forward, embracing the wisdom of Robert Urich's words. A healthy outside indeed starts from the inside, and the holistic approach you've taken in this handbook will ensure that your inner well-being radiates outwards. Together, we'll step into the realm of graceful aging and beyond, a stage where we discover the true beauty of a life well-lived during and after menopause.

INTERACTIVE ELEMENT: YOUR MENOPAUSE SUPERFOODS AND HERBAL REMEDIES SHOPPING LIST

As you embark on your journey to master menopause with grace, here's a handy shopping list to help you stock up on the superfoods and herbal remedies we've discussed in this chapter. Remember, these are tools you can incorporate into your daily routine to empower your menopausal experience. Feel free to choose the ones that resonate with you, and use herbal remedies only if you desire. Your well-being is in your hands, and you have the power to customize your menopausal journey.

Superfoods

- flaxseed
- leafy greens (e.g., kale, spinach, Swiss chard)
- cold-water fish (e.g., salmon, mackerel, sardines)
- prunes
- dark chocolate
- kimchi—or other fermented foods like kefir and sauerkraut
- maca

Herbal Remedies—Optional

- black cohosh
- red clover
- dong quai
- kava
- Korean ginseng
- horny goat weed
- hops
- St. John's wort
- valerian
- soy isoflavones

Feel free to explore these holistic tools at your own pace, and remember that it's always a good idea to consult with a healthcare professional before starting any new herbal remedy or supplement. Your journey through menopause is unique, and by customizing your toolkit with these superfoods and herbal remedies, you're taking the first step toward a more empowered and graceful experience.

8

AGE GRACEFULLY IN THE SECOND COMING OF AGE AND BEYOND

It's time to delve into the profound journey of aging and the wealth of wisdom that accompanies the second coming of age. Menopause is a transformative period in a woman's life, and with it comes a unique opportunity to embrace the full spectrum of your experiences.

Have you ever wondered why I chose to name my eight-step tool MENO-WISE? The answer lies in the essence of this chapter. MENO-WISE isn't just a catchy acronym; it embodies the very spirit of this phase. I called it that because the second coming of age brings a new sense of wisdom. It's about recognizing that menopause is not an endpoint but a new beginning, an opportunity to nurture and celebrate the wisdom that age has bestowed upon us.

In the pages that follow, we will explore the final stage of MENO-WISE, which stands for continued wisdom, menopause management, relentless empowerment, and the endless joy this phase of your life can bring. This chapter is your guide to navigating the journey of aging with a deep sense of empowerment. Together, we will unravel the secrets to making the second coming of age a time of transformation, enlightenment, and unparalleled joy.

So, are you ready to embark on this empowering journey, exploring the wisdom and joy that the second coming of age can bring? Let's dive into the heart of MENO-WISE, discover its facets, and learn how to embrace this remarkable phase of life with open arms.

FIBROIDS SHRINK, CONFIDENCE SOARS, AND INNER STRENGTH RETURNS

As we embrace the second coming of age, it's important to recognize that menopause ushers in a multitude of positive changes that can significantly impact your confidence and inner strength. One remarkable transformation is the shrinking of uterine fibroids, a condition that often affects women during their reproductive years. Let's explore how this physical change can have a profound impact on your self-assurance and your ability to embrace the wisdom that age brings.

Increased Confidence

The reduction in fibroids is not just a relief from physical discomfort; it's a boost to your self-esteem. With the shrinkage of these growths, many women report feeling more comfortable in their bodies. The relief from pain, heavy menstrual bleeding, and bloating can enhance your self-image and allow you to embrace your body's changes with a newfound confidence.

Inner Strength Returns

Menopause is a time when many women rediscover their inner strength. The physical changes, such as fibroid shrinkage, often mirror the emotional and mental growth that comes with age. This phase encourages self-reflection and personal growth, allowing you to harness the inner strength that may have been overshadowed during earlier stages of life.

A New Beginning

Menopause is not the end of your journey; it's the beginning of an exciting new chapter. You can reinvent yourself and explore your true desires and passions, free from the distractions and limitations that fibroids or other reproductive issues may have imposed on you. This is your opportunity to embark on a journey of self-discovery and personal fulfillment.

Aging on Your Terms

Menopause empowers you to age on your own terms. It's a time to redefine beauty and wellness in a way that feels authentic to you. The societal pressures of youth no longer hold the same weight, which allows you to celebrate the unique, meaningful journey of aging gracefully.

Initiating the Wise Woman Within

Menopause initiates the wise woman inside of you. It's a transformative period that encourages you to tap into the deep well of wisdom and experience that age brings. With the physical changes, such as fibroid shrinkage, you're able to fully embrace this wisdom, recognizing the strength and resilience that have always been a part of you.

This phase of life is a celebration of your inner and outer transformation. As you journey through menopause and the second coming of age, you have the opportunity to let your confidence soar, your inner strength shine, and your unique wisdom flourish. You can age gracefully and authentically, free from the burdens of reproductive issues and societal expectations. It's time to embrace the remarkable woman you are becoming, empowered by the wisdom of age and the endless possibilities that lie ahead.

MAINTAINING PHYSICAL AND MENTAL HEALTH: BUILDING RESILIENCE AND ADAPTABILITY

As you progress through the menopause and post-menopause stages, maintaining your physical and mental well-being becomes an essential part of embracing the second coming of age. To achieve this, it's crucial to build resilience and adaptability, which are skills that can help you navigate the changes and challenges that this transformative period brings. In this final step of the MENO-WISE journey, we'll explore what resilience is, what defines it, and how you can continue the positive habits you've adopted in the first seven steps to become more resilient and adaptable.

But first, what is resilience?

Resilience is the ability to adapt and bounce back when life takes an unexpected turn. It's the strength within ourselves that allows us to face adversity, uncertainty, and the various challenges that mid-life, including menopause, might present. Resilience isn't about avoiding difficult situations; it's about embracing them with courage, maintaining our equilibrium, and continuing to thrive.

This phase of life is marked by several factors that can test your resilience. Physical changes, such as hormonal fluctuations and the effects of aging, can challenge your body's adaptability. Emotional and mental shifts, including mood swings, anxiety, and sleep disturbances, might challenge your inner strength. Additionally, the societal expectations and perceptions of aging can sometimes clash with your own self-image and goals, making it crucial to maintain a resilient mindset.

Resilience is defined by your capacity to

- Adapt: Resilient individuals have a flexible and adaptable mindset. They can adjust to changing circumstances and find new strategies to overcome obstacles.
- Bounce back: Resilience enables you to recover from setbacks. Instead of dwelling on failures or difficulties, you learn from them and move forward with a renewed sense of purpose.
- Maintain emotional well-being: Resilience helps you manage stress, anxiety, and negative emotions effectively. It allows you to stay emotionally balanced even in the face of adversity.
- Cultivate self-confidence: Resilient individuals have a strong belief in their own abilities. This self-confidence empowers you to tackle challenges with determination.
- Build support networks: Resilience involves reaching out to friends, family, or professionals for support when needed. Building a strong support system is an essential component of resilience.

- Embrace change: Resilience allows you to see change as an opportunity for growth rather than a threat. You can adapt to new situations with curiosity and optimism.

As you continue the habits you've adopted in the first seven steps of MENO-WISE, it's time to become more resilient and adaptable. Embrace the challenges of menopause and postmenopause as opportunities for personal growth and transformation. With this, you'll maintain your physical and mental health, allowing you to age gracefully and find enduring joy in this remarkable phase of life.

BECOMING RESILIENT: NAVIGATING MENOPAUSE AND BEYOND WITH GRACE

The journey of aging gracefully, especially during the second coming of age and beyond, is not just about enduring the changes—it's about thriving in the face of them. To become resilient and embrace this transformative phase of life with grace, consider the following steps:

Knowledge Empowers

Knowledge is your most potent tool in navigating menopause and postmenopause. Keep empowering yourself with more knowledge and tools for managing this transition. Understanding the physical and emotional changes helps you approach them with a sense of control and empowerment.

Symptoms Are Never Insurmountable

Remember that your menopause symptoms, while challenging, are never insurmountable. By acknowledging that these changes are a natural part of the aging process, you can face them with resilience and a positive mindset. Your ability to adapt to these symptoms and find effective solutions is a testament to your strength.

Sleep Hygiene and Relaxation

Continue practicing good sleep hygiene and relaxation techniques. Remember that a good sleep is crucial. By maintaining a sleep routine and incorporating relaxation methods into your daily life, you can manage stress and ensure your body and mind are in harmony.

Hormonal Balance Routine

Establish a hormonal balance routine that extends beyond postmenopause. Hormones play a significant role in how you feel and function. Maintaining a balanced approach to hormone health can contribute to your overall well-being and resilience.

Enjoy Physical Activity

Continue enjoying exercise and activities that motivate you. Physical activity not only supports your physical health but also contributes to emotional well-being. Engaging in activities you love can bring you enjoyment and pleasure, adding to your resilience.

Keep Your Tribe

Building a support network is vital during this transformative period. Surround yourself with a community of friends, family, and like-minded individuals who understand and encourage your journey. These connections are invaluable in helping you navigate the ups and downs of menopause.

Embrace Change and Stay Positive

Lastly, grow comfortable with change and maintain a positive outlook. Change is a part of life, and your ability to embrace it with optimism can enhance your resilience. As you transition through menopause and beyond, remind yourself of the opportunities that lie ahead and the wisdom that age brings.

Becoming resilient during the second coming of age and beyond is a journey of self-discovery and empowerment. By adopting these practices, you can address this transformative phase with a deep sense of inner strength. Your resilience will not only help you endure the changes but also thrive in a life filled with wisdom, joy, and endless possibilities.

DISCOVERING ESSENTIAL RESOURCES FOR YOUR MENOPAUSE JOURNEY AND BEYOND

It's essential to have access to valuable tools and resources that can support and empower you throughout this transformative journey. Here, you will find a collection of excellent resources, from podcasts and webinars to apps and toolkits, designed to provide you with knowledge, guidance, and inspiration.

Menopause Podcasts

- *CIPD Menopause Podcast:* Tune in to insightful episodes that provide you with a wealth of information, advice, and stories to ease your transition through menopause.
- *Dr. Louise Newson Podcast:* Delve into Dr. Louise Newson's podcast, offering expert insights and discussions about menopause.

Fit and Chips' Chats

Explore *Fit and Chip's Chats* for information on managing various aspects of menopause, including stress and weight gain. These engaging discussions provide practical tips and advice.

CIPD Menopause in the Workplace Webinar

Gain valuable insights into managing menopause in a work setting. This webinar offers guidance for individuals and organizations experiencing the menopause transition.

My Menopause Center

Explore the My Menopause Center's collection of incredible tools and resources designed to empower you with knowledge and support for your menopause journey.

Menopause Preparedness Toolkit

SWHR Menopause Preparedness Toolkit: Download this comprehensive toolkit, *A Woman's Empowerment Guide*, to equip yourself with practical strategies and resources for navigating menopause with confidence.

MENOPAUSE APPS

- Dr. Louise Newson's Balance App: Consider using the Balance App, created by Dr. Louise Newson, to access expert advice, support, and tracking tools to help manage your menopause symptoms effectively.

- Health & Her App: Explore the Health & Her app, which offers an array of resources and community support for women experiencing menopause.
- MDedge: Access this mobile health app, designed to assist women and clinicians in managing menopausal symptoms and promoting overall well-being.

These resources provide a wealth of information, support, and inspiration to help you address menopause, build resilience, and embrace life beyond this transformative phase. Feel empowered, informed, and confident as you continue on your journey of aging gracefully.

In the immortal words of Thomas Fuller, "All things are difficult before they are easy." These words deeply resonate as we approach the conclusion of our journey through the *Menopause Empowerment Handbook*. I want you to remember this: The path to age gracefully in the second coming of age and beyond may indeed seem challenging at times, but this very difficulty paves the way for a more effortless and fulfilling part of your life.

CONCLUSION

As we've traversed the steps of MENO-WISE, you've gained knowledge, wisdom, and a profound sense of empowerment. You've learned to navigate change with grace, embracing the transformative power of menopause. Recognize the incredible achievement that is making it through this empowering journey, for you deserve acknowledgment and praise.

Menopause is a significant chapter in a woman's life. While it is often accompanied by physical and emotional challenges, it is also a time of tremendous growth and self-discovery. The MENO-WISE framework has been our guiding light, helping us understand and embrace the changes that come with this natural transition.

MENO-WISE taught us to be present in the moment and pay attention to our thoughts and feelings. By cultivating mindfulness, we learned to accept the changes happening in our bodies and minds. This self-awareness set the stage for the transformative journey ahead. It empowered us with knowledge. We delved into the science of menopause, understanding the hormonal shifts, physical symptoms, and psychological changes that occur. This knowledge helped us break free from misconceptions and fears, allowing us to approach menopause with a more informed and open mind.

This tool showed us how a well-balanced diet can alleviate many of the symptoms associated with menopause. We learned about the importance of nutrients like calcium, vitamin D, and omega-3 fatty acids. Nourishing our bodies with the right foods became a form of self-care, making us feel more energetic and resilient.

Moreover, MENO-WISE encouraged us to maintain a positive outlook on life. We realized that our thoughts and attitudes could greatly influence our experience of menopause. By focusing on the possibilities and opportunities this transition brought, we cultivated a sense of hope and resilience.

Now that we've completed this journey, it's time to wrap things up and move forward. Your life, filled with knowledge, wisdom, and endless possibilities, is waiting for you. Menopause has equipped you with the tools to face the world with newfound strength and grace. The second coming of age is a time for you to define on your own terms, free from societal expectations and stereotypes.

Embrace this next chapter of your life with open arms, for it is a time when your unique strengths and qualities will shine. The world is ready for the remarkable woman you have become. You've gained resilience, self-awareness, and a deep sense of purpose throughout this journey. Your wisdom and life experiences have molded you into a force to be reckoned with.

So, take a moment to reflect on your journey through MENO-WISE. Recognize the courage it took to confront the changes, the strength required to embrace them, and the wisdom that emerged from this transformative process. You've not only grown as a person but also inspired others along the way.

As you move forward, remember that endless possibilities are awaiting you. Whether it's pursuing a new passion, traveling to new places, deepening your relationships, or simply relishing in the freedom of self-expression, your life is yours to shape. Menopause is not an end but a remarkable beginning.

Let the adventure of the second coming of age begin with enthusiasm and anticipation. With the knowledge and wisdom you've gained, you're well-equipped to navigate the challenges and seize the opportunities that come your way. Embrace this new phase of life as a time of self-discovery, growth, and fulfillment. MENO-WISE has been your guide, companion, and source of strength through the transformative journey of menopause. You've learned to be mindful, educated, and optimistic about this natural phase of life. You've nourished your body, taken care of your wellness, celebrated your identity, and expressed your experiences. Most importantly, you've embraced the changes that menopause has brought into your life.

Now, it's time to celebrate the remarkable woman you've become. Take the knowledge, wisdom, and empowerment you've acquired, and use it to shape the next chapter of your life. The world is eager to see the remarkable things you'll achieve. The second coming of age is a time of limitless potential, and it's yours for the taking. So, go forth with grace and strength, for the adventure is yours to embrace.

As we come to the culmination of this transformative journey through this book, it is my deepest hope that you've found inspiration, strength, and a renewed sense of empowerment in the face of this significant life transition. Menopause is not the end but rather a powerful beginning, where you have the opportunity to embrace change. This concluding chapter is all about summarizing the key takeaways from this book and leaving you with a powerful call to action supported by a heartwarming success story.

In the heart of this handbook lies the message that menopause is a natural and powerful phase of a woman's life. It's not something to be feared or endured but celebrated and embraced. It's a time to regain your confidence, redefine your identity, and welcome the wisdom that comes with age.

But before we finish, I'd like to share a beautiful story about my dear friend Sarah. She was someone who went through menopause before I began my research, and her experience served as a powerful source of inspiration for this book.

Sarah embraced the wisdom found in these very pages and thrived during her second coming of age. She dedicated herself to understanding the changes in her body and mind, taking charge of her health through regular exercise and a balanced diet. She found solace in meditation and surrounded herself with a network of supportive friends who shared her journey.

Most importantly, Sarah used the tools and strategies outlined in this handbook to enhance her emotional well-being and open up about her struggles with her partner. Instead of seeing menopause as a roadblock, she and her husband saw it as an opportunity to rekindle their intimacy and share a deeper, more profound connection than ever before.

As she moved through menopause, Sarah also discovered her true passion: painting. This creative outlet not only brought her immense joy but also redefined her sense of identity. Sarah found that her life was far from over; in fact, it was just beginning.

So, dear readers, as you come to the end of this book, I invite you to reflect on your own journey through menopause. Embrace the powerful message that it's your second coming of age, a time to celebrate your wisdom, body, and life.

Every moment of this phase is an opportunity for growth and transformation. Find joy in the small victories, and don't be too hard on yourself. Menopause is a process, not a destination.

Remember that there will be challenges along the way, but remember that you have the tools and knowledge to manage many aspects of menopause. Take control of your well-being, and seek support when needed.

Not every remedy or strategy will work for every woman. Experiment, explore, and adapt to find what works best for you.

And remember, your story is valuable. Whether you've just started your menopausal journey or have already made significant progress, share your experiences. By doing so, you provide inspiration and support for other women.

I'd love to hear about your journey and how this book has helped you. Please leave a review or comment, and let's continue the conversation. Your feedback and experiences are not only a source of inspiration for me but also a valuable resource for others who are navigating their own second coming of age.

In closing, I wish you the most graceful, empowering, and beautiful second coming of age. If you haven't started this journey, please do. Embrace the wisdom, embrace the change, and discover the amazing potential that lies within you. Life is an adventure, and menopause is just another exciting chapter. Here's to a future filled with grace, empowerment, and endless possibilities.

REFERENCES

Adulted. (2022). *Meditation Techniques to Help with Menopause Symptoms.* Stripes. https://iamstripes.com/blogs/mental-health/meditation-techniques-to-help-with-menopause-symptoms

All Points North. (2022, November 11). *The 5 Types of Intimacy Every Healthy Relationship Needs.* All Points North. https://apn.com/resources/5-types-of-intimacy/#:~:text=SOCIAL%20INTIMACY

AMC Team. (2016). *Talking About Menopause With Friends and Family.* Menopause Centre. https://www.menopausecentre.com.au/information-centre/articles/talking-about-menopause-with-friends-and-family/#:~:text=Own%20it.%20Don

Athey, C. (2023, January 11). *How to bridge the menopause retirement gap in your business.* Boolers. https://boolers.co.uk/how-to-bridge-the-menopause-retirement-gap-in-your-business/#:~:text=Professional%20financial%20advice%20can

Balance App. (n.d.). https://www.balance-menopause.com/balance-app/

Barton, N. (2022). *Navigating menopause as an initiation into your wise woman.* Base Formula. https://www.baseformula.com/blog/menopause-wise-woman#:~:text=I%20recently%20interviewed

Betts, J. (2021). *100+ Inspirational Family and Friends Quotes.* LoveToKnow. https://www.lovetoknow.com/quotes-quips/relationships/60-inspirational-family-friends-quotes#:~:text=

Brown, M. J. (2022, January 21). *11 Natural Ways to Reduce Symptoms of Menopause.* Healthline. https://www.healthline.com/nutrition/11-natural-menopause-tips#calcium-vitamin-d

Can Menopause Cause Anxiety or Depression? (2019, November 25). Cleveland Clinic. https://health.clevelandclinic.org/is-menopause-causing-your-mood-swings-depression-or-anxiety/#:~:text=A%3A%20Unfortunately

Cappelloni, L. (2012, February 15). *Hair Loss and Menopause.* Healthline. https://www.healthline.com/health/menopause/hair-loss

Caring for your skin in menopause. (n.d.). AAD. Retrieved October 30, 2023, from https://www.aad.org/public/everyday-care/skin-care-secrets/anti-aging/skin-care-during-menopause#:~:text=this%20-could%20worsen.-

Castrillon, C. (2023). *Why It's Time To Address Menopause In The Workplace.* Forbes. https://www.forbes.com/sites/carolinecastrillon/2023/03/22/why-its-time-to-address-menopause-in-the-work place/?sh=59a4c6bb1f72

Chen, K. (2019). *An app to help women and clinicians manage menopausal symptoms.* mdedge. https://www.mdedge.com/obgyn/article/202304/menopause/app-help-women-and-clinicians-manage-menopausal-symptoms

Christian, E. (2021, July 13). *5 tips for nurturing friendships during menopause.* Rest Less. https://restless.co.uk/health/healthy-body/5-tips-for-nurturing-friendships-during-menopause/#:~:text=While%20feeling%20snappy

Cognitive Restructuring: Decatastrophizing (Worksheet). (n.d.). Therapist Aid. https://www.therapistaid.com/therapy-worksheet/decatastrophizing/cbt/none#:~:text=Cognitive%20distortions%20are

Colino, S. (2023, June 20). *Herbal Remedies for Hot Flashes, Other Menopausal Symptoms.* EverydayHealth. https://www.everyday health.com/menopause/promising-supplements-for-menopausal-symptoms/#:~:text=study%20found%20that%20women

Contributors, W. E. (2023). *Sex and Menopause.* WebMD. https://www.webmd.com/menopause/sex-menopause

Coveney, P. (2021, June 12). *How Can Yoga Manage Your Menopause?* The Menopause Charity. https://www.themenopausecharity.org/2021/06/12/how-can-yoga-manage-your-menopause/#:~:text=can%20help%20manage

Davidson, J. M. (2023, May 21). *8 Ways to Even Out Menopause Mood Swings.* EverydayHealth. https://www.everydayhealth.com/menopause-pictures/ways-to-even-out-menopause-mood-swings.aspx#:~:text=Chronic%20stress%20can

Debice, S. (2019). *Does The Menopause Affect Friendships?* Inspired Health. https://inspiredhealth.co.uk/blogs/the-menopause-blog/does-the-menopause-affect-friendships#:~:text=This%20is%20a

Deering, S. (2023, August 24). *50 Empowering Quotes About Mental Health for Comfort and Support*. Woman's Day. https://www.womansday.com/health-fitness/wellness/a44901046/mental-health-quotes/

Does mindfulness help with menopause? (n.d.). Balance. Retrieved October 30, 2023, from https://www.balance-menopause.com/menopause-library/does-mindfulness-help-with-menopause/#:~:text=Mindfulness%20body%20scan

Donsky, A. (n.d.). *Family Support During Menopause*. Morphus. Retrieved October 30, 2023, from https://wearemorphus.com/blogs/relationships/family-support-during-menopause#:~:text=Going%20through%20menopause%20can

Dresden, D. (2017, May 22). *Mood swings during menopause: Causes and treatments*. Medical News Today. https://www.medicalnewstoday.com/articles/317566

8 Mindfulness Exercises That Also Reduce Stress. (2019). Hawaii Pacific Health. https://www.hawaiipacifichealth.org/healthier-hawaii/live-healthy/8-mindfulness-exercises-that-also-reduce-stress/#:~:text=One%20of%20the

8 Surprising Facts About Menopause and Perimenopause. (2023, April 24). *Live Healthy*. https://livehealthy.muhealth.org/stories/8-surprising-facts-about-menopause-and-perimenopause#:~:text=Between%2020%25%20and%2040%25%20of%20women%20experience%20depression%20around%20menopause

Eilber, K., Kerrigan, S., Kreps, A., & Madsen, M. (2023). *The Best Menopause Apps to Empower Women*. Doctorpedia. https://www.doctorpedia.com/channels/the-best-menopause-apps-to-empower-women/#:~:text=Caria

Escobar, S.- N. (2023, April 6). *11 Superfoods for Menopause*. Menopause Better. https://menopausebetter.com/superfoods-for-menopause/#:~:text=Maca%20root%20is

5 Self-Care Tips for Thriving Through Menopause. (n.d.). The Women's Center. Retrieved October 30, 2023, from https://www.wcorlando.com/blog/5-self-care-tips-for-thriving-through-menopause#:~:text=Don

Gordon-Barnes, C. (2014, October 12). *6 Fresh Ways to Find Your*

Passion. The Muse. https://www.themuse.com/advice/6-fresh-ways-to-find-your-passion

Grant, M. D., Marbella, A., Wang, A. T., Pines, E., Hoag, J., Bonnell, C., Ziegler, K. M., & Aronson, N. (2015, March 1). *Introduction*. NCBI; Agency for Healthcare Research and Quality (US). https://www.ncbi.nlm.nih.gov/books/NBK285446/#:~:text=Longitudinal%20studies%20have

Hailes, J. (2018). *Menopause & herbs*. Jean Hailes. https://www.jeanhailes.org.au/health-a-z/natural-therapies-supplements/menopause-herbs#:~:text=female%20flowers%20of

Harper, J., Phillips, S., & Biswakarma, R. (2022). *An online survey of perimenopausal women to determine their attitudes and knowledge of the menopause*. NCBI. https://www.ncbi.nlm.nih.gov/pmc/articles/PMC9244939/#:~:text=A%20study%20in%20the%20UAE%20found%20that%2067%25%20of%20women%20had%20poor%20knowledge%20of%20the%20menopause%2C%209%20and%20a%20study%20of%20220%20UK%20women%20found%20that%20women%20had%20little%20formal%20menopause%20education

Harvey, B. (2023, May 31). *71 Best Resilience Quotes for Bouncing Back*. Good Good Good. https://www.goodgoodgood.co/articles/resilience-quotes#:~:text=

He, G. (2022, September 8). *39 Best Work-Life Balance Quotes for Job Satisfaction in 2023*. Team Building. https://teambuilding.com/blog/work-life-balance-quotes#:~:text=I

Herbal Remedies for Menopause, Menopause Information & Articles. (n.d.). The North American Menopause Society. https://www.menopause.org/for-women/menopauseflashes/menopause-symptoms-and-treatments/natural-remedies-for-hot-flashes#:~:text=Kava

Hinsliff, G. (2023, January 12). Not just hot flushes: how menopause can destroy mental health. *The Guardian*. https://www.theguardian.com/society/2023/jan/12/not-just-hot-flushes-how-menopause-can-destroy-mental-health#:~:text=A%20survey%20of

Home. (n.d.). My Menopause Centre. https://www.mymenopausecentre.com

Home. (n.d.). My Systers. https://mysysters.com/#:~:text=myCalendar%20symptom%20tracker

Hooper, S. C., Marshall, V. B., Becker, C. B., LaCroix, A. Z., Keel, P. K., & Kilpela, L. S. (2022). Mental health and quality of life in post-menopausal women as a function of retrospective menopause symptom severity. *Menopause, 29*(6), 707–713. https://doi.org/10.1097/gme.0000000000001961

horm2287. (2018, December 10). *10 ways to combat menopause mood swings*. Hormone Health. https://hormonehealth.co.uk/10-ways-to-even-out-your-menopause-mood-swings#:~:text=Some%20research%20suggests%20the%20herbal%20remedy%20St%20John

Hot flashes - Symptoms and causes. (2018). Mayo Clinic. https://www.mayoclinic.org/diseases-conditions/hot-flashes/symptoms-causes/syc-20352790

Hot Flashes: What Can I Do? (2021). National Institute on Aging. https://www.nia.nih.gov/health/hot-flashes-what-can-i-do#:~:text=suited%20for%20you.-

How to have great sex during menopause and beyond. (2021, May 14). Nebraska Medicine. https://www.nebraskamed.com/womens-health/how-to-have-great-sex-during-menopause#:~:text=Talk%20with%20your

Husband's Guide to Great Sex After Menopause. (2010, October 5). MyVMC. https://www.myvmc.com/lifestyles/husbands-guide-to-great-sex-after-menopause/#c20:~:text=Sexual%20feelings%20change

INFO. (n.d.). Menopause Support. Retrieved October 30, 2023, from https://menopausesupport.co.uk/?page_id=60#:~:text=%25%20of%20women%20experienced%20three%20or%20more%20severe%20symptoms

Jack, C. (2022). *10 Ways to Help a Partner During Menopause | Psychology Today South Africa*. Psychology Today. https://www.psychologytoday.com/za/blog/women-autism-spectrum-disorder/202203/10-ways-help-partner-during-menopause#:~:text=3.%20Talk%2C%20talk

Joshi, S., & Vaze, N. (2010). Yoga and menopausal transition. *Journal of Mid-Life Health, 1*(2), 56. https://doi.org/10.4103/0976-7800.76212

Kopf, J. (2022). *7 Celebrities Who Have Talked Openly About Menopause.*

Health Central. https://www.healthcentral.com/condition/menopause/celebrities-menopause

Losing love for my job... (n.d.). Hellocaria. https://hellocaria.com/losing-love-for-my-job/#:~:text=I%E2%80%99m%20not%20sure,Selma%2C%20New%20Jersey

Luckie, S. (2023, September 8). *How to manage opportunity and promotion during menopause.* We Are The City. https://wearethecity.com/how-to-manage-opportunity-and-promotion-during-menopause/#:~:text=Recognising%20what%20you

Macleod, M. (2021, August 24). *Menopause and flexible working options.* Menopause Training Company https://menopausetrainingcompany.com/menopause-in-the-workplace-what-is-flexible-working-and-what-options-can-you-offer/#:~:text=Part-time%3A

Marinaki, A. (2023, March 24). *150 Best Motivational Quotes To Empower Yourself In 2023.* Email Marketing Automation Platform for Thriving Businesses. https://moosend.com/blog/best-motivational-quotes/#:~:text=

Mayo Clinic Staff. (2023). *The reality of menopause weight gain.* Mayo Clinic. https://www.mayoclinic.org/healthy-lifestyle/womens-health/in-depth/menopause-weight-gain/art-20046058#:~:text=Move%20more

Menopause. (2021). Mental Health Foundation. https://www.mentalhealth.org.uk/explore-mental-health/a-z-topics/menopause#:~:text=antidepressants%20and%20menopause-

Menopause. (2022). World Health Organization. https://www.who.int/news-room/fact-sheets/detail/menopause#:~:text=The%20importance%20of

Menopause: Age, Stages, Signs, Symptoms & Treatment. (2021, October 5). Cleveland Clinic. https://my.clevelandclinic.org/health/diseases/21841-menopause

Menopause and flexible working options. (2021, August 24). Menopause Training Company. https://menopausetrainingcompany.com/menopause-in-the-workplace-what-is-flexible-working-and-what-options-can-you-offer/#:~:text=Part-time%3A

Menopause and Retirement. (2014, February 7). Red Hot Mamas. https://

redhotmamas.org/menopause-and-retirement/#:~:text=If%20you%20have%20a

Menopause and your mental wellbeing. (2022). NHS Inform. https://www.nhsinform.scot/healthy-living/womens-health/later-years-around-50-years-and-over/menopause-and-post-menopause-health/menopause-and-your-mental-wellbeing#:~:text=psychological%20impacts%20of

Menopause Facts, Advice and Support. (n.d.). The Menopause Charity. https://www.themenopausecharity.org

Menopause Fact Sheet. (n.d.). Self Care Forum. https://www.selfcareforum.org/menopause/#:~:text=Mood%20problems%20and

Menopause in 2022: Addressing a knowledge gap. (2022). Cuyuna Regional Medical Center. https://www.cuyunamed.org/wellness/menopause-2022-addressing-knowledge-gap#:~:text=There%20is%20a

Menopause Preparedness Toolkit: A Woman's Empowerment Guide. (2022, June 16). Society for Women's Health Research. https://swhr.org/swhr_resource/menopause-preparedness-toolkit-a-womans-empowerment-guide/

Menopause resources. (n.d.). CIPD. Retrieved October 30, 2023, from https://www.cipd.org/uk/topics/menopause/#:~:text=Webinars

Menopause Self-Esteem. (2023). Meno Martha International Menopause Directory. https://menomartha.com/health-topic/menopause-self-esteem/#:~:text=

Menopause Support and Resources | Hormone Health Network. (n.d.). Endocrine. https://www.endocrine.org/menopausemap/support-resources/index.html

Menopause—Support networks for menopausal women. (2018). Health Talk.org. https://healthtalk.org/menopause/support-networks-for-menopausal-women#:~:text=Organised%20support%20groups%0ASome

Menopause: the benefits of acupuncture. (2018, March 27). Physiothérapie Universelle. https://physiotherapieuniverselle.com/en/blogue/menopause-benefits-acupuncture/#:~:text=Acupuncture%20helps%20restore%20the%20body

Menopause - Things you can do. (2022, May 24). NHS. https://www.nhs.uk/conditions/menopause/things-you-can-do/#:~:text=exercise%20regularly%2C%20including

Menopause wellbeing: how to set goals to boost your health and happiness. (2022) Balance. https://www.balance-menopause.com/menopause-library/menopause-wellbeing-how-to-set-goals-to-boost-your-health-and-happiness/#:~:text=plans%20and%20coping

Mindfulness-based stress reduction (MBSR) - MBSR exercises. (n.d.). Guy's and St Thomas' NHS Foundation Trust. Retrieved October 30, 2023, from https://www.guysandstthomas.nhs.uk/health-information/mindfulness-based-stress-reduction-mbsr/mbsr-exercises#:~:text=All%20of%20the

Mishra, N., Devanshi, & Mishra, V. (2011). Exercise beyond menopause: Dos and don'ts. *Journal of Mid-Life Health, 2*(2), 51. https://doi.org/10.4103/0976-7800.92524

Mitchell, G. (n.d.). *The Importance of Self-Care.* Menopause Centre. https://www.menopausecentre.com.au/information-centre/articles/the-importance-of-self-care/#:~:text=So%2C%20what%20does

Mitchell, G. (2020). *How Personal Boundaries Can Improve your Life.* Menopause Centre. https://www.menopausecentre.com.au/information-centre/articles/how-personal-boundaries-can-improve-your-life/#:~:text=Here

Mohamad Ishak, N. N., Jamani, N. A., Mohd Arifin, S. R., Abdul Hadi, A., & Abd Aziz, K. H. (2021). Exploring women's perceptions and experiences of menopause among East Coast Malaysian women. *Malaysian Family Physician, 16*(1), 84–92. https://doi.org/10.51866/oa1098

Mohsin, A. (n.d.). *How Does Menopause Impact Sexual Desire?* Progressive Women's Health. https://www.progressivewomenshealthonline.com/blog/how-does-menopause-impact-sexual-desire#:~:text=Some%20women%20experience%20an%20increase

Montgomery, T. (2023). *Embracing Ageing On Your Terms: Redefining Beauty in Midlife.* LinkedIn. https://www.linkedin.com/pulse/embracing-ageing-your-terms-redefining-beauty-midlife-montgomery/#:~:text=Ageing%20is%20a

Murphy, J. (2016). *How menopause stress can impact relationships*. Saga. https://www.saga.co.uk/magazine/health-wellbeing/mind/ menopause-affect-friendships# :

Namazi, M., Sadeghi, R., & Behboodi Moghadam, Z. (2019). Social Determinants of Health in Menopause: An Integrative Review. *International Journal of Women's Health, 11*, 637–647. https://doi.org/ 10.2147/ijwh.s228594

Our purpose. (n.d.). My Menopause Centre. https://www.mymenopause centre.com/our-purpose/#:~:text=We

Page, S. (2022). *57 Quotes on Wellness and Health to Inspire Healthy Living*. Total Wellness Health. https://info.totalwellnesshealth.com/blog/ quotes-on-wellness-and-health#:~:text=

Perry, S. (n.d.). *Keep Calm: 7 Ways to Strengthen Your Resiliency*. Prime Women. https://primewomen.com/wellness/build-resiliency/#:

Perimenopause: Age, Stages, Signs, Symptoms & Treatment. (2021). Cleveland Clinic. https://my.clevelandclinic.org/health/diseases/21608-perimenopause

Posadzki, P., Lee, M. S., Moon, T. W., Choi, T. Y., Park, T. Y., & Ernst, E. (2013). Prevalence of complementary and alternative medicine (CAM) use by menopausal women: A systematic review of surveys. *Maturitas, 75*(1), 34–43. https://doi.org/10.1016/j.maturitas.2013. 02.005

Postmenopausal Bleeding: Causes, Diagnosis & Treatment. (2021). Cleveland Clinic. https://my.clevelandclinic.org/health/diseases/21549-postmenopausal-bleeding

Postmenopause: Signs, Symptoms & What to Expect. (2021, May 10). Cleveland Clinic. https://my.clevelandclinic.org/health/diseases/21837-postmenopause

Preparation Quotes. (n.d.). BrainyQuote. https://www.brainyquote.com/ topics/preparation-quotes#:~:text=The%20best%20prepara-tion,Jackson%20Brown%2C%20Jr

Rose, H. (2022, December 1). *Self-Care for Menopause: How Can You Help Yourself*. Calmerry. https://calmerry.com/blog/self-care/self-care-for-menopause-how-can-i-help-myself-during-menopause/#:~:text=Try%20acts%20of

Santen, R., & Loprinzi, C. (2023). *Patient education: Non-estrogen treat-*

ments for menopausal symptoms (Beyond the Basics). UpToDate. https://www.uptodate.com/contents/non-estrogen-treatments-for-menopausal-symptoms-beyond-the-basics/print#:~:text=SSRIs%20

Sexy Ageing Blog Posts. (2023). Sexy Ageing. https://www.sexyageing.com/pages/blog-site?p=body-image-and-menopause-an-ongoing-saga#:~:text=Focus%20on%20Health

Sleep Problems and Menopause: What Can I Do? (2021). National Institute on Aging. https://www.nia.nih.gov/health/sleep-problems-and-menopause-what-can-i-do#:~:text=To%20improve%20your

Spritzler, F. (2021, May 12). Tips for Losing Weight Around Menopause (and Keeping It Off). Healthline. https://www.healthline.com/nutrition/lose-weight-in-menopause

Sreenivas, S. (2023). Birth Control During Menopause. WebMD. https://www.webmd.com/sex/birth-control/birth-control-during-menopause

Sweet, W. (2019, February 28). Best Relief For Menopause - Natural Treatment & Remedies. My Menopause Transformation. https://www.mymenopausetransformation.com/success-stories/#:~:text=When%20it%20comes

Sweet, W. (2023, March 1). The road to resilience for women in perimenopause. My Menopause Transformation. https://www.mymenopausetransformation.com/womens-health/the-road-to-resilience-for-women-in-peri-menopause/#:~:text=exercise%20or%20activity

10 Best Resources to Support Your Perimenopause and Menopause. (n.d.)| menopause-ology.com. Menopause-Ology. Retrieved October 30, 2023, from https://menopause-ology.com/10-best-resources-to-support-your-perimenopause-and-menopause/#:~:text=Fit%20n

10 Quotes on Overcoming Obstacles That Will Motivate You. (2023, August 5). Teamphoria. https://www.teamphoria.com/10-quotes-on-overcoming-obstacles-that-will-motivate-you/#:~:text=

The Emotional Roller Coaster of Menopause. (2023). WebMD. https://www.webmd.com/menopause/emotional-roller-coaster

Theobald, M. (2014, December 4). 7 Winter Superfoods for Menopause

Symptoms. EverydayHealth. https://www.everydayhealth.com/ pictures/winter-superfoods-menopause-symptoms/#:~:text=Fish%20that%20thrive

Towers, I. (n.d.). *Reframing Ageing this Women's Health Week: Embracing Our Beauty Beyond Menopause.* International Towers. Retrieved October 30, 2023, from https://www.internationaltowers.com/ whatson/reframing-ageing-this-womens-health-week-embracing-our-beauty-beyond-menopause#:~:text=the%20Hill%20or

Triiyo. (2022). *Top 8 Tips to Prepare Your Finances for Retirement.* LinkedIn. https://www.linkedin.com/pulse/top-8-tips-prepare-your-finances-retirement-triiyo/#:~:text=Reassess%20your%20lifestyle

Upham, B. (2023, May 23). *10 Reasons to Look Forward to Menopause - Menopause Center.* EverydayHealth. https://www.everydayhealth. com/menopause-pictures/positives-of-menopause. aspx#:~:text=Increased%20Confidence%20and

Vaginal Dryness: Causes & Treatment. Cleveland Clinic. (2022). https:// my.clevelandclinic.org/health/symptoms/21027-vaginal-dryness

Waichler, I. (2023). *Menopause & Depression: Connections, Signs, & How to Cope.* Choosing Therapy. https://www.choosingtherapy.com/ menopause-depression/#:~:text=can%20be%20difficultto%20try%20to

whitecoat. (2020, May 29). *8 Ways to Practice Self-Care During Menopause.* Chapel Hill Gynecology. https://chapelhillgynecology. com/ways-to-practice-self-care-during-menopause/#:~:text=7.%20Stay%20Connected

Wild, S. (2023). *What's the best exercise for the menopause?* bupa. https:// www.bupa.co.uk/newsroom/ourviews/menopause-exercise#:~:text=aspect.%20This%20means

Women's Behavioral Health: Perimenopause Services at UPMC in Central Pa. (n.d.). UPMC Life Changing Medicine. Retrieved October 30, 2023, from https://www.upmc.com/services/south-central-pa/women/services/behavioral-health/conditions/peri menopause#:~:text=Perimenopause%20refers%20to

Yogasana For Menopause: 5 Praiseworthy Yoga Poses To Provide Relief From

The Associated Symptoms. (2023). Netmeds. https://www.netmeds.
com/health-library/post/yogasana-for-menopause-5-praisewor
thy-yoga-poses-to-provide-relief-from-the-associated-
symptoms#:~:text=the%20heart%20rate.-

www.ingramcontent.com/pod-product-compliance
Lightning Source LLC
Chambersburg PA
CBHW051257250726

48656CB00004B/1338